Mommy, I Feel Sick

Mommy, I Feel Sick

DR. CLAIR ISBISTER

Consultant Pediatrician, Royal North Shore Hospital
Sydney, Australia

HAWTHORN BOOKS, INC.
Publishers/NEW YORK
A Howard & Wyndham Company

MOMMY, I FEEL SICK

Portions of this book were published originally in Australia under the title *Mummy, I Feel Sick*.

Library of Congress Catalog Card Number: 77-99076

ISBN: 0-8015-5116-1

1 2 3 4 5 6 7 8 9 10

Contents

Mommy,
I Feel Sick

1
Illness in Childhood

There have been so many changes in child care in recent years that parents must wonder if the child specialists are playing tricks on them. It was not so very long ago that you were being told to train your children early; then there was "Let them decide when they are ready. Don't frustrate their little egos." Now it is "Set limits appropriate to the child's stage of development." In other words, don't get tough until the child is over five years of age, but if you don't say then what is expected, the world will give the child a hard time.

When I was just a young, enthusiastic pediatrician starting practice, a mother taking her two-year-old to the hospital would have had the child taken from her at the ward and then firmly but kindly told "No, we don't want any toys. You may come and visit for an hour next Sunday afternoon." Your feeble protests that Bobby loved his teddy bear and would miss his father and mother would have been countered with "It only upsets children to see their parents; he won't miss you. In a few hours he will have settled in nicely and be perfectly happy. His teddy bear will only carry germs and probably get lost, so don't leave it." This still does happen in some places, but now most hospitals allow parents to visit sick children every day, and doctors emphatically tell parents that they must spend as much time as possible with the sick child. There are even militant parent groups making life very difficult for the nursing staff by disorganizing the whole hospital routine and demanding their rights. I saw one incident recently where an entire family of at least three generations asserted their right to have a birthday party in the ward for their two-year-old relative and arrived fully equipped for it.

I am sure, too, that your mother and grandmother get some surprises when they look into your medicine cupboard. What has happened to the castor oil, the liniments, the poultices, the Epsom salts, the Tiger Balm, or whatever miracle ointment was the family favorite? Most parents are well aware from *Readers Digest*, *Time*, the women's magazines, TV, and the news that there have been wonderful advances in medicine; in fact, many parents expect instant cures. But do you all know about the work being done all over the world by children's specialists, psychiatrists, and psychologists in studies of normal children and their needs? What are the most important influences in their lives? Do you know what their fears are and what they think about when they are sick?

Illness is very disturbing emotionally

For all of us, illness is a stressful experience. For children it can be a damaging one that leaves its marks throughout life. Children are nature's reason for our very existence; they are our stake in the future; they *are* the future; they should have the best we can give them, yet the sad fact is that neither we nor the experts know just what is the best for them. As Margaret Mead says, "Things are happening to our children that should never be allowed to happen." However, we are steadily increasing our knowledge, and those who work with sick children appreciate very acutely how much there is still to learn about their needs.

Children's wards are always the most cheerful in the hospital, because the children themselves are such wonderful little patients—no self-pity, no petty complaints, and an amazing ability to fit in and accept what comes—most of the time, anyway. But we often fail to realize how they feel about it all. Just because they seem good and quiet we used to think all was well; now we know that many children get nervous upsets, that illness is very disturbing emotionally, and physical illness may be prolonged by fear and anxiety. Studies of children's needs point to one outstanding need, love—parents' love for them and their love for their parents, on which security, happiness, and their very lives may depend. These are such powerful influences that it has become obvious we cannot separate any child, no matter how well adjusted, from any sort of parents—no matter how bad—without some emotional reaction.

Some very interesting research done in institutions has led us to believe that the longer the separation and the younger the child, the more lasting and disturbing the effects. Well, obviously, there are occasions when children must be separated from parents. There are serious illnesses and operations that need special nursing and medical attention. There are mothers who simply do not know enough to nurse even a mildly sick child at home and mothers who are working and can't afford to lose their jobs. There are good mothers and bad mothers, but it is also a fact that very few of us are able to nurse our own

desperately ill child. The mere fact that we are anxious
and afraid makes us bad nurses, so let us not go to extremes and feel that our physical presence is all that matters. We know that parents can transmit emotions to
young children; in fact, it even seems that discord between
the parents may disturb the child more than separation
from them; you may well help your child and yourself
most by quietly sitting by the bed and letting the nurses
do the nursing.

What of the changes in visiting hours? Well, a minor
revolution has occurred; parents, nurses, and doctors are
getting together better. The hospitals where daily visiting
has been tried report that the children are happier, they
get better quicker, they have fewer nervous reactions and
fewer infections. The parents are happier and the nurses
like it better because they see their little patients as real
people, members of a family, not mere cases in bed, and
this improves their nursing efficiency. There are still some
diehards who sit in offices and shake their heads, but the
people who work in the wards know that this is a great advance in the care of sick children. It raises its own problems. But more of them later.

Treat the whole child

Let us now look more carefully at some of the changes
that have occurred in medicine in the last ten years. One
big change, as I have mentioned, has been the increasing
awareness of the child's mind and feelings. We now try to
treat the whole child, not merely a disease of the body. We
accept the World Health Organization's definition of
health as "complete mental, social, and physical well-
being, not mere absence of disease." This positive ap-

proach has caused many changes. We can no longer give a
bottle of medicine for constipation, flatulence, or vomiting
if we suspect that the cause lies in the mind and the
emotions. The bottle of medicine will still help, but we
must go deeper. There are still doctors who only concern
themselves with the physical aspects and there are still patients who only want the magic in the bottle, but they are
disappearing.

Once I was in the butcher shop when an old man hob-
bled in, leaning heavily on his stick. The butcher said,
"How's your knee, Dad?" "Gettin' better," he replied,
"but it's a bit slow. I'm still takin' those pills the doctor
gave me back in May '67, but they seem a bit slow. Do you
think they're gonna work?" Even the old-timer is beginning to doubt the medicine's efficacy, or at least think a
change of pill is indicated. Medicine in the bottle is being
consumed in greater quantities than ever before, but it
does not work the way it did in the old days when the doctor used to look at the bottle and say, "You missed two
doses last week; see you take it all next week," and the patient got better from an illness that he never dared ask the
doctor to explain. The educated public of today must
know more about their illnesses, though it does not always
help them; they are now beginning to realize that the way
they live, the job they do, the food they eat, and the
thoughts they think all vitally affect their health.

Magic in the bottle

But do not misunderstand me: There is still plenty of
magic in the bottle, more wonderful magic than ever before—penicillin, sulfa drugs, a wide spectrum of antibiotics, serum to prevent poliomyelitis, diphtheria and

typhoid, cortisone and other steroids, amazing anesthetics, and sedatives. They demonstrate the incredible magic of the scientists, but none of them cures disease. They alter the balance of power, but it is nature that restores the damaged tissue to normal. We give drugs to kill germs, we cut out diseased organs and even replace some with transplants or artificial ones. We supply missing vitamins, hormones and enzymes, but we only help nature to restore the situation to normal, and we should never forget that we are aiming for normal according to nature.

The advances in the care of physical diseases are almost unbelievable. There are blood transfusions, antibiotics, anesthetics that make possible the most complicated heart and lung operations, ways of feeding people through their veins, even artificial hearts that can be used during operations. It is possible to save the lives of thousands for whom death was inevitable ten years ago and to prevent illness that was unavoidable for our parents.

But it is all so scientific! There is so much new knowledge that no one person can learn it. Heart and chest operations need highly skilled surgeons, who often do these operations and no others. There are specialists for nearly every organ, and the more each specialist knows about his own speciality the less he knows about everyone else's. Between you and these highly skilled men is the general practitioner. Many of our general practitioners in Australia have served a year as resident doctors in a children's hospital, or teaching hospital with a children's ward, and have considerable knowledge of the diseases of children, but there has arisen a special sort of general physician, the children's doctor, or pediatrician. These doctors have received special training in development and diseases of children, spent several years working in children's hospitals, and have taken specialized training in child health. Some pediatricians practice as general practitioners who see only children, and the more highly qualified and senior ones as consultants only. General practitioners call in the pediatrician for the more unusual and difficult problems of child care. Each age has its own problems of growth and development, and pediatricians are unique in that they specialize in an age group rather than an organ. They all have appointments at hospitals where they care for children, and every big hospital now has its pediatricians.

Admission to the hospital

The need for specialized care, specialized nursing, specialized medicine, and surgical techniques has made it absolutely impossible to care for the more serious conditions at home and still give the child all that medicine now has to offer. That is why we have decided that since it hurts children to separate them from their parents, then their parents must come to the hospital. We have learned that much can be done to relieve the mental stress of illness. Increased visiting by parents is far from all; some parents are anything but soothing, and they have much to learn about the child's needs. Many hospitals do not give the patient a very encouraging reception. How would you like to be asked your name, address, and religion, whether you can pay the bill (or even to make a down payment), and then be told to have a bath before you even get near a bed? It is much worse for a child to have all his clothes whisked off by a strange woman and his mother packed off until next Sunday! No, we doctors admit that we have a lot to learn about admission to the hospital, and we are trying. If we are to get the best results, parents, nurses, and doctors must cooperate and learn as much as they can about the reactions of the child and how to help.

Love

The younger the child, the greater the need for the every-day world. Babies are still almost part of their mothers; they do not know where they end and their mother begins. They notice the difference when other people handle them. They may become lonely and confused. We know that there is a stage they reach if kept in the hospital for a long time without a mother substitute when they cease to gain weight, become pale and listless, and slip back. They sometimes used to die by sheer wasting away, but if we allocate nurses to particular patients so that they really get to know each other and encourage the mother to come frequently and take over some of the nursing, a transformation occurs. What medicine is this? *Love*, the greatest power of all in helping children back to health, and we have to learn to use it. Though the mother usually does most of the day-to-day care of children and her influence is the greatest in the early years, research shows that the father is just as important. The child wants to see him just as much, and as a rule, he will be greeted with more enthusiasm than the mother.

Many years ago the psychiatrist, John Bowlby, said "What is believed to be essential for mental health is that the infant and young child should experience a warm, intimate, and continuous relationship with the mother or permanent mother substitute in which both find satisfaction and enjoyment," but more recently he said, "There is a strong case for believing that unthinking confidence in the unfailing accessibility and responsiveness of attachment figures is the bedrock on which a stable, self-reliant personality is built." The father is an important attachment figure. Books such as *Early Experiences* by Clark (Open

Books Publishing) and *Mothering* by Rudolph Schaffer (Fontana) reviewed the literature. They draw attention to the quality of relationships between parents and their relationship with their children and the balance between masculine and feminine principles in the cherishing of children.

When young children under three come into the hospital they react in several ways. The very sick are usually too sick to care much about anything, and they will often sleep peacefully with a parent sitting beside them. The majority of children make quite a fuss when the mother first leaves, then they gradually settle down and accept the situation. Some become quiet and seem to retire into themselves, some appear hostile, some fret and cry continuously; these last have more than normal emotional reactions to this experience. There may be some psychological problems in the family relationships (and who doesn't have those sometimes?) or this may be an unusually sensitive child.

Reactions to stress

All children slip back in behavior when they are sick; those who have been dry during the day will have toilet accidents, those who have been eating solid food will only want their milk, and those who have been speaking fluently may keep to monosyllables or simple sentences. Many will try to comfort themselves by some form of bodily stimulation like thumb-sucking, head-banging, rocking, or masturbation. All of these are reactions to stress; they may matter very little and merely indicate the need for more emotional support, or they may again lead the doctor to investigate some management problem at home. We do know that the children who have unusual reactions or emotional difficulties are usually already having difficulties at home, and an observant nurse and doctor get a wonderful opportunity to help sort out more than the mere physical illness. We all have our own pet ways of behaving under stress; the important thing as far as these sick children are concerned is to reduce the strain while in the hospital, not try to reform their habits then and there. Daily visiting under medical supervision, improved admission arrangements, and better preparation for the hospital will make a big difference to the mental health of the child and consequently to physical health.

Minor operations

We know that some children, more than others, need their parents, and what disturbs one child will not disturb another. Many minor operations that used to be done early are now delayed until the child is over three years of age and by then they have often been found to be unnecessary. For instance, the operation of circumcision used to be regarded as almost a necessity for newborn boys but now pediatricians look on it as rarely necessary, a matter of preference and religious belief. Even then it is much less frequently done in the hospital when the child is newborn, more liable to infection, and has barely accommodated to life. It is left till he is a few weeks old. Hernias of the navel are now left till over three years of age in most cases; by then the majority have cured themselves. Adenoids and tonsils are not whisked out the way they used to be; a safe rule, for tonsils at least, is not under five years of age without the serious consideration of the specialist, particularly in allergic families. Of course, all these operations are essential in some cases but not as often as it was formerly thought, so doctors can reduce the need for admitting children to the hospital. If mothers learn more about nursing their children we can keep the hospital for the children who really need it. All the recent advances in mental health are stressing that doctors, nurses, and parents must know more about the needs of children.

2
Johnny's in the Hospital

The modern practice of encouraging parents to visit their sick children daily if they can, and even in some cases to have the mother live in the hospital, was primarily to relieve the child of the emotional stress of separation from parents. It has, however, had some other very valuable results; it has proved a wonderful opportunity for mothers to learn more about nursing sick children so they can look after them better and perhaps keep them at home during their next illness. It allows parents, too, to see the kindness and the untiring efforts of the hospital staff, so that difficult parents often turn over a new leaf. It has made the hospital staff more conscious of children as people, improved communication between staff and parents, and raised the general standard of patient care.

Parents

Do not imagine that I am overly sentimental about parents. Being one, I know how it feels to have a child in the hospital, but I have had the experience of difficult, almost impossible parents whose children would fare better away from them forever, parents whose one idea seems to be that the whole world wants to defraud them and neglect their child, parents who plague one's life with minor complaints, and parents who insult us by offering to pay large sums of money if we can hasten the child's recovery or save its life and finally refuse to pay the most moderate account. But the child has to live with these people, loves them, and in their own inadequate way they return that love. An interested doctor can often see ways to help both parent and child. There are parents who abuse the hospital authorities because their child is not completely recovered upon return home. Parents are the trial of every doctor's life, but those of us who have our own children know the agony that parents suffer when their child is ill.

If the visits to the hospital merely teach some of the elements of hygiene, then we have done some good. I remember one mother who was asked to come and give her baby a bottle of milk. She took it and had a quick swig herself first in front of the horrified nurse. She explained that she always tested the milk that way to see if it was too hot. The head nurse walked in just at the critical moment and the entire visiting scheme trembled in the balance.

There are times when even good, capable parents are better kept away from their children for a little while. We want parents to help remove fear and give the child a feeling of security; weeping, terrified parents cannot do this; if they cannot conquer their fear (and it is a very difficult thing to do), it is better for them to rely on a cheerful, confident nurse. The child's whole world topples when the parents, who mean protection and security, are obviously afraid. There are times, too, when even the excitement of seeing the parents may be undesirable. The doctor and nurses must decide this.

Some helpful suggestions for parents

There are a few points that may help parents when they visit the hospital. Visitors should be limited to those who mean most to the child, usually the father and mother, but should include the person who is familiar, such as grandma or mother's helper, if she has one. Too many people in the wards at once excite children and spread infection, so explain tactfully to your friends and relatives that the daily visiting does not apply to them. If a mother cannot visit her under-five-year-old daily, then it would be beneficial to leave packages with the nursing staff or send a card each day. One mother I know left a little parcel to be opened as soon as she left and that removed the distress of good-bye; others have left parcels or cards to be opened each day, and others have given the child a toy telephone to keep in touch with mommy. A toy telephone and the four-year-old's imagination do wonders.

How the child will react to your visit

Direct all your questions to the nurse in charge of the ward or your child's doctor. Do not ask junior nurses or passing doctors; you may get confusing answers. Find out the best time to visit; find out if the child can have candy, fruit, ice cream, etc. Never give them without asking, as it can be very distressing to have to take them back from a sick child. Ask if you may help feed the patient. Read stories, try to be yourself, and act as you would if you were caring for the child at home. Find out if you are allowed to cuddle the ill child, but do not expect a normal reaction toward you. The two-year-old may feel let down and even

deserted by the mother, and may "freeze" and perhaps refuse even to recognize you. Some mothers get so upset that
they think the child has forgotten them, but even babies do
not forget! The child's feelings have been hurt and must be
won back patiently and lovingly. In such instances the ill
child may be openly hostile or cling frantically, refusing to
let the mother go. Mothers should try to take it all quietly
and lovingly.

What to bring

The child will almost certainly yell when you leave, but
don't let that worry you. Give a warning shortly before
you have to leave, perhaps pointing out the place on the
clock where the hand has to be when you must go. When
the time comes to depart, go promptly; do not prolong the
harrowing moment. A good, protesting yell is soon over
and does much less harm than the misery of no visit. In
any case, when the child discovers the next day that you
really come back, things will not be so difficult. Be cheerful yourself and listen to all the child has to tell about the
hospital doings, or just sit quietly if that is what is wanted.
Please do not bring things that cause a mess, like modeling
paste and chalks; bring things that are appropriate for the
child's age—a few colored blocks for an eighteen-month-
old, a cheap book of big, brightly colored pictures for a
two-year-old, tiny cars for boys from three to ten, dolls for
little girls who just love dolls to dress and undress and play
with. Remember, it is the child who has to be satisfied, not
our philosophy. Avoid easily broken toys or that will be
another heartbreak for a sick child. By all means bring
strong, hard-wearing toys, not too many, and label them

with the name of the child. Do not let them accumulate; even the best nurses will not be able to keep track of them, so do not bring in any valuable toy. Let the child have a favorite old teddy, no matter how decrepit, for it's a link with home. If there is any special toy that is taken to bed, see that it is provided or the child may find it hard to get to sleep. Stuffed toys are dirty things, but when the baby is sick it is no time to take them away. Some mothers feel too ashamed to mention the stuffed toy, and we wonder why the child lies awake or won't stop screaming.

Your visit is very important, but it must be done the child's way. You have come to make the hospital feel a little more like home. Play with and feed the child, be natural, don't scold or criticize, or let on that you disapprove in any way of the treatment.

Preparation for the hospital

We often find that children have quite the wrong idea about the hospital, and many of their fears could have been prevented by better preparation. What, then, can parents do about this?

Even the bravest of us get a sinking feeling in the pit of the stomach when we have to go to the hospital. It is a strange place, strange bed, strange food, often noisier than home, and medicine and needles are often unpleasant. Well, it is stranger still and more frightening for children. But you can help them. You can bring up your child to regard doctors and nurses as kind people who make sick children better. You can take your child to see the local hospital when an opportunity arises and let him become familiar with nurses' uniforms, wards, and doctors' white coats, even at the age of two. Tell the child about little

Johnny, who was sick and went to the hospital, and the doctors made him better. Don't make it sound like a holiday and don't make it frightening, but make sure that everything you say is the truth without giving too much detail.

Nurses now get lectures in child development and child psychology, as well as lectures on the diseases of children. I often wish there were a syllabus of lectures that all parents had to take, but there does not seem to be much chance of that. One has to be trained for every career except the two most important: governing the country and rearing its future citizens. Socrates said that long before I did, but it is still true. Extraordinary, isn't it? Perhaps these subjects are too controversial for training, but a wider knowledge of the essential needs and of child behavior could not go astray.

Parents' attitudes

Most parents do love their children and try to do their best for them, but they do say some strange things and make life very difficult for us physicians if they do not tell the child the truth. My pet abominations are the mothers who say, just as the doctor is about to give an injection, "The doctor won't hurt, dear," or "Stop kicking or I'll tell the doctor to cut your legs off with the big knife he has." Then there is the mother who leaves her child in the hospital and says, "I'll be back in a minute; I'm just going outside," and then does not come back for a week.

How can these children feel secure? Lies like that leave the child feeling alone, terrified, and trusting no one. If the child grows up with the general idea that most people need treatment in a hospital for their own good at some time, and that illness is unpleasant and the hospital makes it better, then you won't go far wrong. If, however, a child hears you discuss Uncle Bill's hernia that went wrong, and Aunt Mary's agony when she had her operation, you can't expect belief that the hospital will help, particularly if the child has also overheard the details of Aunt Mary's funeral. Little pitchers indeed have big ears. Incidentally, it is also very effective propaganda to allow the child to overhear, apparently accidentally, the reverse type of conversation about how well Uncle Bill was treated and how he had an awful pain and the nurse gave him something that fixed it so quickly. Children are more alert than their elders in detecting propaganda, so be truthful, remembering that you are preparing the child to face an actual experience.

Children have vivid imaginations. There is no need for detail, except perhaps about toilet arrangements and meals. Try to keep the whole talk impersonal and not let the child realize that this is preparation against the day of admittance. It is like sex education. If you give too much detail and relate it to the child, you overemphasize it and make the situation apprehensive. There are a number of good books about hospitals, too, which help to make children familiar with the idea of what a stay there will be like. Dressing carts, food carts, the operating theater and ambulances are just as interesting subjects for conversation for four-year-olds as snails, garbage trucks, fork lifts, cranes, and the origin of our milk supply, all of which may be discussed in the course of any day. But there needs to be as little emotion as possible about it all.

When you have forewarning about admission to the hospital, it is just as well for the child to know that at some time there will be an operation. The child then gets a chance to get used to the idea, to learn that an anesthetic is simply a sleep that stops pain, and that soreness afterward will occur. The actual day should be kept secret until near the day of admission: the younger the child, the shorter the notice. The poor little eighteen-month-old child just has to go without notice, and as with all other ages when things happen suddenly, you must just give the child support and stay nearby as much as possible. When children have to go to the hospital unexpectedly, as is so often the case, then don't try to cram in all the information you feel you should have given them; it will only make them anxious and you can repair your failure during visiting hours.

Home from the hospital

What about when the child comes home from the hospital: Are there problems then? It was the frequency of behavior problems after an illness that first drew the attention of doctors to the fact that children were often disturbed by illness and the hospital. So many mothers came back with the story that the child had been spoiled in the hospital, that the child clung to her skirts and cried whenever she left the room, that nightmares, bed-wetting, masturbating or excessive thumb-sucking were the norm. The child of two who, deep inside, blamed mommy for what happened because she had been the main protector, may be a very difficult little person on coming home, may refuse to have anything to do with her, may really set out to annoy her, may run away, but most often makes quite sure that she will never, never, never go out of sight again. This child becomes a persistent and adherent little shadow until the mother is nearly crazy. But can you blame such a reaction?

Is it surprising that, after having had penicillin injections in the night or having heard other children having them, the child will wake and scream in anticipation? Is it surprising that the child will not go to bed? There was enough of bed in the hospital, and at times the nights were more than a little frightening. You can expect some troublesome behavior; you may be able to think the way the child thinks and see why it is happening. There is not much that will not respond to firm, sympathetic handling and patience, but you may be helped by having a talk with the doctor or nurse in charge of the ward. You may unearth something that is worrying the child and about which a five-year-old merely needs reassurance. I know one little girl who had a nightmare at the same time every night until her mother discovered that it was the time the child had been given her penicillin shot in the hospital; her mother told her that there would be no more needles and that was the end of the trouble—dramatic as that! So don't be surprised if, for a few nights, the child wants the light on or you to sit alongside until sleep comes.

Remember that children's behavior always means something to them. If you push away the clinging child or smack the hostile one, you are really confirming suspicions that you don't love the child any more. If you get the child occupied with something in the room where you are working and accept the fact that you must not be out of sight unless the child chooses to leave you, and if you can provide distraction rather than hit back, this phase will soon pass and the child will realize that your love and protection still obtain. Children's emotions are no more mature than their bodies; love and hate are primitive affairs, easily aroused, and if the mother behaves in a primitive fashion without the adult virtues of gentleness, patience, and understanding, then she is in for trouble.

The first week home from the hospital is not easy. The child is usually demanding, not eating well, and feeling poorly, so you have to be prepared to give up time at the expense of the house, the rest of the family, and certainly your social engagements.

3
Home Nursing Made Easy

Does your child need to go to the hospital?

Sick children do need good nursing and often specialized medical care, but I hope I haven't frightened you into thinking that you are not capable of looking after your own ailing child. All pediatricians prefer to keep the sick child at home as long as as the home conditions are satisfactory and the mother able and willing to do the nursing patiently and thoroughly. As I have often said before, we pediatricians prefer to avoid worrying or frightening a sick child, and regarding most fevers children get, we find they subside quicker at home.

This means that every mother should know the essentials of home nursing—how to wash a sick child, how to take a temperature, how to make the child comfortable in bed, how to prepare simple food, and a few tricks about how to get medicine down. I think perhaps, too, mothers need to know a few danger signals, but on the whole, I find mothers are very alert to the changes in their child's condition and soon let the doctor know if they are worried. It would really be a good idea to join the Red Cross. If you

24

just learn a few of these points in nursing care perhaps you will feel more confident that you are doing the right thing when you are looking after a sick child.

First a word of caution: Do let your doctor decide whether your child needs to go to the hospital. I have seen a mother take a seriously ill child from the hospital because she insisted that the child needed her more than anything else in the world, when what the doctor thought was most needed was some intravenous feeding at once. She endangered the child's life because she had an unbalanced outlook; she could have stayed and sat beside the child, but that wasn't enough. Important as a mother's love and comfort is, it cannot replace expert nursing and medical care when they become necessary. If you feel quite sure you are capable of looking after your child and the doctor is quite sure admittance to the hospital is called for, then it is a matter for the father and mother to discuss with the doctor. It often happens that the doctor knows you can look after the child, but is afraid important signs of change will be missed. Very often we pediatricians don't know what is wrong when the child first runs a high temperature. We don't want to rush in with treatment that may be unnecessary, yet we feel a nurse won't miss a new symptom. We like to feel that a trained person is watching, so please accept your doctor's decision.

Does the child really need to go to bed?—Well, not all the time, anyway. In the feverish stage it is best, but you must have the child near so that you can hear every call. Sick children get very upset if their calls are not heard or if they are kept waiting. They cry and that makes them very tired and blocks up their noses so that they feel unhappier still. You certainly must not go out of earshot of a very sick child. This usually means putting the child on a couch in the living room if you want to get any housework done, or staying in the bedroom when the child is awake, unless ringing a bell is acceptable. The trouble then is that it is apt to be fun to ring a bell for mommy.

The Room: The room should be airy, but not drafty. Usually, opening the window a few inches at the top attends to this, but see that the bed isn't between the door and the window. Remove everything that harbors dust; sweep and dust the room before you move the child into it, or preferably vacuum-clean it. Dust is very irritating to the child with even a mild cough, and children are funny little creatures; they don't complain about things like dust, or cold, or heavy bedclothes, or crumbs in the bed. You have to find out what might be uncomfortable for them. So don't shake up pillows or blankets in the room, and do see that the bedding is not too heavy. It's no use putting thick, heavy bedding over little children; the weight tires them and they often throw off the covers and get cold. It's much better to see that they are warmly clad. Put a cardigan over their pajamas if necessary, and put socks on, then it doesn't matter if they push off the coverings. You can always slip something over them when they get off to sleep. That is when they need covering most.

The Bed: The child must be comfortable. The mattress should be firm. An inner spring, good kapok, or rubber one is fine. Don't have one that is so soft the child sinks into it. Chldren tend to sweat a lot because their temperature goes up and down a lot more readily than that of adults. They will be very uncomfortable, and on a soft mattress, get sweat rashes easily. Give the child one smallish pillow to lie down on, or three to be propped up against. It is hard to get comfortable on two. For the under-three-year-olds, put an oilskin raincoat, rubber sheet, or piece of plastic between the sheet and mattress. I know it's hot, but it's not so bad if you have a piece of blanket or an old comforter to cover it, and it saves a lot of washing.

Little ones who have had perfect control of bowels and bladder when they were well, have accidents when they are ill, particularly if their bowels are loose. This is very distressing to the child, who hates that kind of mess. Be sure you have a bedpan or a wide-based bottle within easy reach for all ages, though it's wise to have that oilskin also.

Vomiting is another difficulty you can anticipate. Most young children with a fever vomit, whatever the cause. It's a messy, smelly, uncomfortable business that the child hates, and a towel over the side of the pillow in readiness saves a lot of washing. Often there is not time to reach the basin you have left close by (or even to lean over the side and be sick on newspaper, as some people recommend), whereas the child will grab the towel, and a towel is a lot easier to wash than a sheet and a blanket. Cover the bed with a washable spread and see that the sheet is turned down well over the blanket.

Even if you manage to avoid the dirtied beds and spilled glasses of water that most of us have to contend with, you will probably find that you need to change the bed linen more than usual, particularly the pillowcase which is soaked with perspiration. Soiled linen should be removed immediately and stains dealt with before they dry (see the end of chapter under *Stains*). A bed is always more comfortable and warmer if it is made with an underblanket between the bottom sheet and the mattress. Be sure you have all the things you need to make the bed before you start, then see that the bottom sheet is pulled firm and tucked in well to avoid creases. A child can usually be placed in a chair wrapped in a blanket while you make the bed, but can be put back when you have the bottom sheet in place. The rest of the bed can be completed then. Tuck in the sheet and blanket firmly at the bottom, but not too tightly across, as you want to allow for a fair bit of movement. See that the bedding is not too heavy. A light, washable nylon or acrylic cover is better than heavy blankets. Then use a washable bedspread over the top. If the child is too ill or too irascible to be moved out while you make the bed, then there is a neat way of making the bed without the move. You get the bottom sheet on one side first, smooth it across and roll the child onto it, then off the other side, tucking in the sheet.

To Wash or Not to Wash: This is a big question. It is more important to keep the bedding and pajamas clean than the child, so don't be too fussy about spotless cleanliness. I think we wash people too much in the hospital and at the most absurd hours. Washing can be very tiring for sick people, though it can be refreshing and pleasant. The important thing is comfort. Obviously, if the child is perspiring a complete bath is required, but if the child has a high temperature and is sleepy, the face and hands may be enough. Certainly never wake a sick child for a bath and never wash the child by force. If you meet resistance, wait until a better time.

When you do wash the child, have everything ready on a table beside the bed, not on the bed—soap, washcloth, bowl of warm water, two towels, and talcum powder. Do the child a little bit at a time, keeping covered the parts not being washed. Before you start, slip a towel under the arm or leg you are going to wash; then you can dry it quickly and gently, and you won't spill any water on the bed. Be sure to dry the child thoroughly, and remember, talcum powder is soothing and refreshing. If the child must be in bed for more than a few days, then use a little methylated spirits. Rubbed on the back they stop infected rashes and bed sores.

A sick child will often fall asleep after having hands and face sponged, and sleep is so important. You will often find that after breakfast you may have just straightened the bed and no sooner sponged the child's face than sleep intrudes. You can leave the child until afternoon for a more thorough bath. But don't worry if you have to leave the child unwashed for a whole day or even two days or more, as long as you can keep the bedding and clothing clean. Don't forget the teeth, however. Children get a dirty tongue and bad breath with most fevers, and their mouth will get dirty, particularly if they won't drink much. Older children will wash out their mouth and brush their teeth, but it isn't always easy with the little ones, so you may have to help.

Normally the mouth and teeth are kept clean by saliva and the action of chewing and swallowing. However, in illness, particularly if the nose is blocked, the child tends to breathe through the mouth so that it becomes dry and the tongue coated. The child may object very much to having either the teeth or mouth cleaned, but may be prepared to chew a piece of apple. Even if it is spat out soon thereafter, it does very nicely.

Brushing hair and cleaning nails are not important, but do become necessary after a day or so and are better done once a day for comfort.

How to take a temperature

I think every mother should be able to take a temperature. I know some fuss and rush to the thermometer unnecessarily, but that is no reason for not being able to use one, and I always feel very exasperated when I meet women who say rather proudly, "I wouldn't keep a thermometer in the house." That's silly. If a mother is nursing a child at home with a fever, then I like her to be able to tell me what the child's temperature is. Children run high fevers easily, often for quite minor reasons, and there is nothing to be unduly alarmed about in a temperature of 103 °F or 39.4 °C with no other worrying symptoms.

The normal temperature is 98.4 °F or 36.9 °C if taken under the arm or in the mouth; it is a degree higher in the bowel. For children under five the safest place is under the arm or in the groin in contact with the skin, but the thermometer must stay five minutes to record accurately. You will usually find it best to sit beside the child reading a story, because five minutes is a long time. For a child over five, place the bulb of the thermometer under the tongue and see that the mouth is kept shut. Breathing through the mouth lets in cold air and keeps the temperature reading down. Most thermometers are supposed to record in half a minute, but they rarely do; one and a half minutes are necessary in the mouth. For taking temperatures in the bowel a special rectal thermometer is needed, and though this is the way we always take a baby's temperature in the hospital I really think it is safer for mothers to keep to the armpit or groin.

Now, once again don't be alarmed by the height of the temperature alone. It does indicate that the child is reacting well, is fighting off infection, and from that point of view it is not worrying. However, most children are very drowsy over 104 °F or 40 °C and some may have convulsions, so it is usual to recommend sponging to get the temperature down a little if it's over 103 °F or 39.4 °C. Sponge the hands, face, and back of the neck with cold water; there is no need to undress the child, but turn back the bedclothes and let the child cool off.

Temperature without Fears: Evening temperatures tend

to be higher than morning, and most people will vary a degree from morning to night anyway. Children's temperatures may fall below normal when they are shocked, as after an accident, or when the temperature has been high and has suddenly fallen, and it is important then to see that they are kept warm. So be on the alert for the cold, clammy skin, and take the temperature if you think the child feels cold, or hotter than before. Actually, it is very hard to guess a temperature by feeling the child's skin with your hand, just as you can't rely on your hand to test the bath water. However, I think the cheek or lips are a fairly good guide, and by holding the child's hand to your cheek or kissing the forehead you can get a good idea of whether a fever is present.

When you take a temperature always be sure to shake down the mercury well below normal first or you will get a false reading. After using, wipe the thermometer with alcohol to clean it; don't on any account run hot water over it. These thermometers are only made for reading body temperatures and they break very easily in hot water. In the hospital we take temperatures at four-hourly intervals, but I think three times a day is sufficient for a child at home with a fever. But do write it down, so that the doctor can see just what is happening. The doctor may also want you to observe the pulse and how fast the child is breathing. These are not easy, but a little practice and any mother should be able to do it.

How to take a pulse

To take the pulse you place three fingers along the wrist at the base of the thumb. You will feel an artery pulsating under your fingers. Count for half a minute and double it to get the rate per minute. Infants under two will normally have a rate between 100 and 140 per minute; children 90 to 100. It goes up if the child cries or struggles, so try to take it during quiet moments. Counting breathing rate is harder. Though normal rhythmical breathing is regular, it varies with emotion, talking, and exercise, and we can consciously alter it by holding our breath, so you have to count breathing when the child is unaware of what you are doing. One breath in and out counts as one breath. A baby may breathe thirty to forty times a minute normally, a child about twenty-five and adults under twenty. It is also important to notice sounds like wheeziness, crowing noises, and coughing.

Now about this problem of bowels and urine. I have said already to have a potty nearby, and for boys, a big, flat-bottomed bottle for urine, so that you can easily see how much is passed and whether it looks normal without making a fuss about it. A fall in the output of urine may be the first sign that a child cannot tolerate a drug or has developed a kidney complication or is simply not taking enough fluid to wash out waste. A child on sulfa drugs must have sufficient fluids or crystals may form causing pain and blockage to the passage of urine.

Mothers always get agitated about bowels, and sometimes I feel doctors these days don't take enough notice. Often the old family doctor of the last generation started his treatment of a child with a fever by ordering calomel or castor oil—both severe, unpleasant, and often dangerous medicines. After that there was a reaction against opening medicines. However, I would make this point— that the bowels are meant to get rid of waste and it should not bank up during illness. A child is very uncomfortable after several days of constipation, so I think it is best to order a mild opening medicine like cascara at the beginning of the fever, provided there is no tummy pain, vomiting, or diarrhea.

Try to avoid the frequent use of soap sticks or suppositories, but when a child is really constipated, say, after four days, a suppository may be less uncomfortable than an opening medicine. The doctor may suggest a small enema. Most mothers would take the child to the hospital to get a nurse to give an enema, but it is not really difficult. The old-fashioned enema was a simple bowel washout using weak salt water—a teaspoon of salt to a pint of a very weak, soapy water mixture. This was run into the bowel slowly through a rubber tube lubricated and inserted gently into the rectum with the child lying on one side. A four-year-old would need about 8 ounces. These days we use little prepackaged enemas done up in plastic containers with their nozzles all part of them so no extra equipment is needed and a much smaller amount is used. Just insert the nozzle, squeeze in the contents, and remove the nozzle. Wait, with a bedpan close by! (For more details on constipation see page 72.)

The seriously ill child is usually easy to handle, but as soon as life becomes even mildly interesting again, irritability sets in. There is nothing for it but to be calm, cheerful, sympathetic, and gentle, and if necessary, just stay alongside the bed. The feverish child sleeps a lot, and when awake has a right to have you nearby. The child may want a story or just company and the security of feeling mommy is near. The same is true of favorite toys. The child may not want to play with them, but usually wants them close at hand. Don't worry about how you are going to clean them. Use an antiseptic solution for the washable ones, and if sunlight isn't enough for the teddy bear, then dry cleaning will help.

It is no time to start worrying about habits like thumb-sucking when a child is ill, so if the child wants to suck on a thumb or on a puppet or an old rug, allow it. The stress of illness often makes little habits worse, but wait until the child is quite well before you start doing anything about them.

You will be amazed, too, how quickly children lose condition; in no time your chubby little boy seems to look like a pale little waif, particularly if he has had some vomiting and diarrhea. Don't worry, he will put on weight nearly as quickly as he lost it, but it does help to see he moves about in bed a bit. That may sound silly to you, since the usual trouble is keeping children in bed at all. But if a child is very sick he will keep very quiet, especially with heavy bedclothes, and it may be necessary to see that his position is changed. The best way of keeping circulation stimulated is just by getting the child to move about a bit in bed. Once allowed out of bed, even in a chair, it is very hard to keep the child in bed at all.

Stains:

Blood—wash in cold water and sponge with weak peroxide solution.

Food—wash in cold water, then in hot soapy water or detergent.

Fruit juice—pour warm water over stain while wet. If dry, soak in weak peroxide solution.

4

What Can the Child Eat? and Medicine Without Tears

Food and medicine are certainly a mother's main worries when her child is ill. In fact, some mothers fuss so much about food that they disturb the child's rest trying to give it. I would say sleep and liquids are more important even than medicine for most feverish conditions. Children should only be wakened for sulfa drugs and antibiotics; other medicine can wait. You may have heard the German proverb: "Sleep to the sick is halfway to health." Well, it's true.

Sleep

Children's sleep varies a great deal. Some children are restless; others sleep so heavily that you will worry whether they are in a coma or not. There are a few points about watching a sleeping child that I think you should know. Color should be a normal pink or sometimes pale, but if there is blueness, especially around the lips, tell your doctor. Watch the child's breathing. It will be faster than usual with any fever (more than twenty inhalations and exhalations a minute) and it will often be shallow. If it gets deeper or uneven or noisy, apart from sniffles, then gently try to rouse the child. It is not unusual for a child to twitch occasionally in sleeping, but if little twitchy movements happen every now and then, the child's temperature may be going up and a sponging may be necessary. It is easy to take a temperature reading when the child is asleep and quite possible to place a wet, cooling towel on the forehead without disrupting slumber.

Food

To come back to food. Sick children can go for days with very little food. They lose their appetite during a fever and their digestion is upset, and no matter how tempting the food looks you are wasting time preparing it if the child doesn't want it. Merely enough water and salt to replace what the child is losing as perspiration, urine, bowel movements, and perhaps vomiting are all that are necessary. The child also needs some sugar for the acute stage. The rest will be made up later, but liquid is important. However, don't think you have to go to extremes and make the child drink pints. A pint to a pint and a half is good for the whole day in the very feverish stage.

Sometimes the child will only drink as much as can be passed in urine, but try to get more down, and of course keep an eye on how much is passed or you may find the child is in trouble. This is particularly true if the child is on sulfa drugs and is not washing out the wastes in urine. Do give the child pleasant drinks: sweetened orange juice, barley water and lemon or orange juice, and milk—iced, colored, and flavored with vanilla or strawberry. Often you will find that flat lemonade will be all the child wants, so don't despise such drinks. There is nothing wrong with them and they are a good way of getting the child to take both sugar and liquid besides giving a nice clean feeling to the mouth. Make up small quantities of liquids and keep them fresh, offering only a little at a time. A big drink will often make a child vomit, and milk with cream on top or frozen orange juice with the water separated on top are very unappetizing. Leave water and soda water by the bed; other drinks should be offered freshly made.

If the child has diarrhea, the doctor will tell you to try to get down some salt. That is quite easily done by putting a pinch in the lemon or orange juice, or better still by making up barley water with a little salt and adding that to the drinks. Taste the mixture yourself and see that you are not offering a nasty, salty liquid that will make the child vomit. Remember: Appetite is apt to be flagging, and if only water is wanted, then be glad of that. Make everything you offer attractive. Milk is a food as well as a liquid, so if the child takes a little of it iced, colored, and flavored with vanilla or tea, then that is very good. You may ask if the child would like fruit or custard or jello, but only bring small helpings. Usually ice cream is the most acceptable food. The appetite for meat and vegetables usually comes back last, so the child may be days on fruit and puddings.

For the baby the best rule is to offer simpler food than usually given. Give the usual milk mixture unless the child has diarrhea, but stop solids and vitamin preparations except for vitamin C. If the child is not having solids, then weaken the milk mixture and wait until hunger indicates that more is wanted.

The child with whooping cough will often vomit straight after the meal and then want more to eat. Let that be, but try to avoid drinks with meals and crumbly things that irritate. Tonsillitis and mumps mean that chewing and swallowing will be painful, so keep to oatmeal or cream of wheat, sloppy foods, and an occasional nonalcoholic eggnog or milk pudding. Remember, anything that smells appetizing is agony for the mumps sufferer, because it stimulates the sore glands to produce saliva. So keep away those nice smells and, above all, lemon juice.

Don't fuss about food or beg the child to eat. None of this emotional "Do it for mommy, darling." No child ever starved to death in the few days of an infectious fever; try giving small helpings. My dear old grandfather, who was never sick, always used to look at a big helping and say, "When I'm better." You need to feel well to tackle a big plateful. Otherwise it puts you off.

Medicine without tears

Most of us have a few pet household remedies, and our favorite opening medicine (not castor oil), but apart from these, do be careful about giving mixtures you have in the house. You may be wrong about the diagnosis, or the medicine may not have kept well. If you give the stuff that fixed dad's flu you may well give the wrong doses. Above all, never give the drugs and antibiotics "on spec"; they may be dangerous. In hospitals we see too many children with blocked kidneys and severe anemia because their parents did not realize the danger of treating with powerful drugs what might have been only a mild infection. You may have a capsule left over from a previous illness and be tempted to use it, but you mustn't. It must be used under medical supervision only.

One thing that often worries doctors about letting a sick child be nursed at home is whether the child really gets the medicine. It is amazing how often parents miss a dose because the child seems better. With antibiotics and asthma medicines—in fact most medicines—it is necessary to keep up a particular level in the blood and a missed dose means the level of the medicine in the blood drops and symptoms start to reappear; worse than that! It may enable a germ to grow accustomed to the antibiotic and it then becomes ineffective. Be sure you measure the medicine correctly and give it according to instructions. Then there is the problem of getting it into the child, but it isn't really so difficult if you go about it the right way. Most medicine can be made palatable and children are very reasonable. There must be no fuss and emotion, everything very matter-of-fact, and no force. Well, not much! No scolding, no threatening.

Try to arrange some activity, like a story, or a reward like a dessert immediately afterward, and don't for a moment let the child think that you expect any resistance. Tablets and drops can usually be mixed in honey or sweetened condensed milk. Liquid medicine goes down best in sweetened condensed milk or fruit juice, but it is wise to choose something that is not a regular article of diet because he will probably take a temporary dislike to it. So don't put medicine in the porridge or pudding. Capsules and hard, shiny pills are difficult for children. Ask your doctor if it is all right to crush them; if not, they may slip down in butter, or the medicine may have to be changed.

Nose drops usually cause chaos, but if you put a pillow under the child's shoulders, get the head well back, lay the child first on one side and then the other, you can get the drops into the nose and sinuses without letting them run down the throat. That is what is really objected to, and the moment the head is lifted, if not done correctly that is what happens.

I often find that one of the big difficulties in nursing

children at home is the conflicting advice that mothers receive from granny and the next door neighbor. I have frequently discovered some treatment that the child was receiving about which I knew nothing, and which was certainly not doing the child any good. Mother was afraid to own up because granny had been so very convincing in her assurance that "this is what cured you when you had croup." Now do be careful about this. No doctor is going to object to a chest rub or liniment, or even a poultice, but tell him and don't be tempted to try some other medicine on the quiet.

There are some medicines that just don't mix without unpleasant results. Some of the new drugs don't act in the same way as those our grandmothers knew. Before antibiotics our best solution was to apply hot foments and get all abscesses to come to a head and break. Now we get them early and clear them away and we don't usually want foments, so it may surprise you very much to know that there are times when it is quite wrong to foment an early boil.

Cough mixtures were used for every cough and cold, but nowadays most doctors use them very little. It is realized that the cough is nature's way of getting rid of discharges that get into the chest and it is better for a child to cough up the stuff; the exception is the dry, irritating cough and the cough that goes on all night. There are soothing mixtures for those, but it would be wrong to use soothing mixtures in the daytime when there is mucus to be got up. There is quite a lot to be said for honey and lemon, and Vicks Vapo-Rub, but the long, complicated cough mixture prescriptions of previous generations are rarely used now. Another new group of drugs, the antihistamines, is used a lot for allergic conditions. Some of these are used in cough syrups.

A thing that can quite easily happen these days is for a doctor to order an antihistamine or a soothing cough syrup (and some of them are powerful), and later find that his patient is getting a double dose because the outpatient doctor or the specialist they saw recently has already given a similar mixture. This can be serious, and I am often surprised to find how mothers will keep on with one doctor's medicine and not tell the second doctor she is using it. I know it isn't on purpose, but when the same child is getting two lots of treatment things can go wrong.

Another silly thing that often happens is for patients to go on taking the medicine until the bottle is finished, regardless of what happens. That always reminds me of the true story about the women who had a heart attack and was ordered to stay in bed until the doctor saw her again. He was very busy and forgot to go back, but four years later he met her daughter and asked how her mother was and was told she was still in bed where he had told her to stay.

Medicines are dispensed in convenient amounts and quite often a little more than necessary, though just as often I suppose a second bottle may be needed. But don't think that just because you get a bottleful it is the correct amount.

Another thing to be careful about is vitamin preparations. We use them a lot these days to help build up general resistance and to replace deficiencies that occur because of our refined diet, and we tend to use powerful concentrates so that fifteen to twenty drops will be the full dose for the day. It is not good to give an overdose, particularly of vitamin D, so if you are using a concentrated drop preparation you must not give cod-liver oil emulsion or cod-liver oil and malt as well. And for goodness' sake don't do what so many people do; that is, take a double dose because you

feel it doing so much good. Vitamins are natural substances, but that doesn't mean they are harmless.

Sleeping tablets and sleeping drafts also need a caution:
These drugs, and there are many of them, have been a
wonderful advance in medicine. But they can be dangerous and some are habit forming, and they should only be
used to assist patients over a temporary difficulty while
either the acute infection or the emotional disturbance set-
tles down. Occasionally, a sedative may be ordered for
mother *and* child while the mother is learning to understand the situation and coming to grips with it. Of course,
it is wonderful to have drugs that will give a sick patient
sleep, that most precious of all treatments. Children vary a
great deal in the dose they need and it is often necessary to
make changes in the quantities needed, so make quite sure
that you ask your doctor the most you can use and how to
work it up if necessary. Don't experiment by yourself and
don't just stick to a dose that isn't doing the job. Ask your
doctor. Don't imagine he is going to be insulted because it
didn't do the trick the first time.

In recent years there has been a tendency to use simpler
prescriptions, more medicines made up by the drug firms,
and more natural medicines such as vitamins, iron, and
diets. Even nose drops, inhalations, and laxatives are
used much less. The standard of medicine has improved.
Doctors don't just order treatment for a cough, or a headache, or constipation. They look over the whole situation
and try to find the cause and treat that, so that at times
you may even feel that what you called the doctor for isn't
being treated. We don't use throat paints for tonsillitis any
more. We usually try to assist the patient to fight off his
own infection.

We also use special tests a lot more than doctors of the
last generation. We realize that it is silly to treat anemia

unless we are quite sure of the cause and for that we need a blood count. It may be dangerous to treat tonsillitis and abscesses without taking a swabbing to grow the germ and find out what drugs will be most likely to cure them. There is much less need for hit-and-miss methods these days. We can be more accurate in our diagnosis with the assistance of the laboratory. So respect the doctor who uses these aids. Ask the doctor what the test is for, what it may show, what use it can be to the child, and when to expect the result. Some doctors order more tests than necessary, and a careful physical examination may avoid some.

5

The Doctor's House Call

Well, how do you choose a pediatrician in the first place? A doctor may be quite a brilliant diagnostician and order all the right treatment, but he is not much use to you if your child dislikes him and you cannot understand what he is talking about. Fortunately, most doctors who choose to do general pediatrics do so because they like children and can make themselves understood by them. Your general practitioner may recommend a pediatrician, friends or neighbors may be satisfied with theirs; otherwise the proof of the pudding may be in the eating. From the parents' point of view, does he explain exactly what he thinks is wrong and the reason for the treatment he is ordering, and does he make sure that you can contact him if you are in trouble? Does he tell you how to prevent the problem happening again and what to do if it is a recurrent problem? From a child's point of view, does he go quietly about the business of finding out what has happened from the parents while the child is allowed to play and explore the new surroundings and get proper bearings? Does he explain to the child what is to happen, talk about the stethoscope and the auroscope and explain what they are for, let the child turn on the light and generally make sure that no

44

lethal instruments are around, usually explaining very early in the proceedings that there will be no needles this time? We always have awful trouble with the children of engineers, because engineering is an exact science and the father always says, "Now exactly what will this medicine do? How long will it take to act? Do we give it before or with or after food?" And on he goes so that I feel that if I say, "I hope the medicine will cure the fever, but I don't know when it will take effect, because your child may absorb it faster or slower or be more sensitive than others, and I don't care when you give it," then I shall probably get the sack, but I might well be telling the truth.

Doctors are not all the same

Some doctors are always emphatic and definite in their instructions and most agree that it is safer to be so. Some will go to a great deal of trouble to explain to you as much as you want. Others consider that explanations confuse people and they just give instructions so that you don't even know what your child is being treated for. Well, don't growl about it; you have the whip hand. You choose your doctor, and it isn't a scrap of use going to a doctor in whom you have no confidence. You have a perfect right at any time to change your doctor, and you have a perfect right to ask for a specialist's opinion. Only a very opinionated doctor will object. He is usually very glad to share the responsibility of worrying patients and have the opportunity of getting a specialist's opinion. However, do remember that you are the loser if you change your doctor often, because no one gets really familiar with your family and their home problems, and a doctor who really knows and understands your family is a treasure indeed.

In these days of group practices, where several doctors work together and relieve each other, it is unavoidable that there will be times when you don't see your own doctor. But there is still a history card.

Count the cost

Medical benefit plans have been a great help to parents who have children. I urge you to join an insurance plan if you are not already covered, as medical expenses can be a great worry and hospital expenses worse still.

There has been a lot of discussion in the papers lately about fees and insurance, and it is quite obvious that there is a lot of unnecessary misunderstanding. Doctors' fees do vary; obviously they must. Some doctors, unlike others, have put in many more years of study in a skilled specialty and have dearly bought experience in years of study and expenses. It is absurd that their time and skill should have the same value put upon them as those of less qualified doctors. So get it all straight yourself. Ask what the cost will be. How are you to know otherwise? The old system of the doctor just lowering his fee for those he felt could not afford it has been forced out by the new scale of fees fixed by insurance plans for certain treatments. In the long run this will be better for everyone, but it does mean that you should study your plan, get to know more about doctors' qualifications, and find out what benefits you are paying for; and do join the plan that allows you pathology and X rays, and a specialist's opinion if necessary, since these will be very expensive items if they prove necessary.

Doctors are making house calls less and less frequently now, as diagnostic and other aids are so much more sophisticated than they used to be and can only be used at the hospital. However, on the occasions that a doctor does come to your home, here are a few points that will save you embarrassment and the doctor's time. You have sent for him because your child is sick, and you usually have time to prepare. Doctors are not miracle workers and they don't practice magic. A good doctor does not walk into the room and announce dramatically after two questions and a prod in the tummy that your child has an acute appendix. Even though he is in a hurry and has half a dozen more calls to do, he is going to ask lots of questions and examine the child thoroughly. He wants to see movements and urine and vomit, and he wants the facts straight. Do not say, "He got his pain the day he went to the zoo," or "He has the same symptoms as Aunt Mary had last year when she had to have sulfa and it brought her out in hives." You have no idea how infuriating and time-wasting this sort of conversation is.

He will want to wash his hands

Don't prepare for the visit by tearing round madly, cleaning the house and removing all evidence of illness. Doctors are understanding people; we see you at your worst, worried, weeping, no makeup, too tired to clean the bathroom, and we don't blame you. But we do blame you if you put your own feelings before your child's health, so think of the child and all the doctor should know about. Of course, as I said, you can save yourself embarrassment by anticipating the doctor's needs. He is sure to want to wash his hands and may need to boil a syringe, though in these days of sterile disposable equipment he may have one ready for use; anyway see that there is soap and a clean hand towel in the bathroom, and the kitchen need not be in quite such chaos if you think ahead.

And if everything is in a mess, what of it? Don't be all embarrassed and apologetic. You aren't trying to sell the house. Be thinking of the questions you want to ask. What can Susie have to eat? Can she have a laxative? How long will she have to stay in bed? How long will she be infectious? How long will she be away from school? Does her medicine have to be at a fixed time and does she have to have it during the night too? Do you have to keep the baby away from her? There are lots of things you will think of as soon as the doctor is out of the door, so please be a cooperative parent, have the story ready, and even a list of questions written down.

When to call the doctor

One question that I find mothers constantly worry about is when the child should be seen by a doctor—not what hour of day but for what reasons. This may mean taking the child to the doctor or to a hospital emergency room if your own doctor does not do house calls. It is a very difficult question to answer, because it depends entirely on the individual experience of the mother. None of us is calm and placid when our children are in trouble; doctors are often the worst because we know the possibilities and call in another doctor to share the responsibility for quite minor troubles. So it is not just a matter of knowing how to nurse a child or how to diagnose an illness. A lot depends on how worried you are and where you live. Some like to have the doctor's help for every cold; others will wait until it is too late, and quite a few do not like to worry the doctor with what may be trifles.

If you are worried, then you have a perfect right to ask for your doctor's help, and no mother should go on treating a child for anything if it is not improving after a couple of days. There are some urgent signs that indicate you should not attempt to treat the child yourself at all: bluish or yellow skin color; rapid, noisy, or distressed breathing; drowsiness where the child is hard to wake; headache with a temperature; any sudden illness that has come on in a few hours; severe pains in the stomach that last more than an hour and cause a feeling of sickness; high fever.

I think, if it is possible, a doctor should see all cases of acute infection, such as measles, mumps, and hepatitis. They all have complications, and quite apart from the need for accurate diagnosis, you will need some advice about management. You don't just say, "Oh, it's chicken pox, it will soon be better." Chicken pox is a nasty, itchy disease that sometimes gets infected.

Asthma and bilious attacks are in rather a different group. The child who gets asthma often does not need the doctor and may feel more confident if it is possible to get through the attack without calling him. Asthma has to be tackled in several ways—breathing exercises for normal use of the chest, relief from psychological strain, discovering if there are substances like house dust to which the child is allergic, and finally by controlling infection. If the child only gets asthma after a feverish cold or chest infection you may need the doctor every time, but if it occurs after a party or playing with the cat, you may learn to anticipate attacks and give the child medication before the exciting event or as soon as he starts to wheeze.

Bilious attacks are often psychological and, of course, often just dietetic indiscretions; if the child has no pain in the tummy apart from the discomfort of vomiting, then wait a while and see what a water and sugar diet does first. Also, be very wary of blaming teething for too much. Children are teething continuously from six months to two and a quarter years, and though some sleep badly and get irritable with pain, they don't run high fevers or continuously refuse food and look miserable without a more serious cause. The numerous skin rashes they get will usually also require medical care, since it is not always easy to decide the cause. You may make a mistake about German measles or impetigo.

6
Complications and Convalescence

During the acute stage the sick child is not really difficult to nurse, but most of your time is occupied because you have to be nearby and you will be worried. The child is easy to deal with, however, sleeping much of the time and taking medicine quite peacefully. It is when the child begins to feel a bit better that your love and patience are taxed to the utmost. You are still expected to come at every call, the child won't stay in bed, asks for food, then won't eat it when you produce it. A plaintive "mommy!" follows you all day long.

When can the child get up?

In these days of antibiotics and sulfa drugs, the period of high fever may be only a day, but even one day of severe illness is exhausting for the little patient (and his mother); the old rule of allowing the child up after twenty-four hours of normal temperature no longer holds if he is still on antibiotics. I am sure that many get up too soon because they seem normal, but the effects of the illness do not wear off as quickly as that. Tonsillitis and middle-ear infections should be given a week to settle. Colds, measles, chicken pox, mumps, and whooping cough still last as long as they used to. We sometimes have the added problem of an allergic reaction to care for. Many children are now sensitive to penicillin and sulfa drugs, so you have to be on the alert for vomiting, swelling (particularly of the face), rashes, such as itchy lumps or pink or purplish blotches, passing less urine than usual and blood in the urine. Some of the antibiotics cause diarrhea and pains in the tummy, and a severe sensitivity reaction can be worse than the original illness. But don't let me frighten you. These drugs are life saving, and as long as you report to the doctor if you have any suspicion that they may be upsetting the child you won't get into trouble. Always find out what the medicine is for, and which bottle is which, so that you give it intelligently and delay the next dose while you find out if it has caused some new symptom.

I have mentioned that we often let the child up too soon; perhaps I should change that, or ask you not to take it too literally. I mean keep the child warm, indoors, warmly clad, and fairly calm. A child is often better off sitting on a rug on a sunny, protected porch than leaping all over the bed in a cold bedroom. Also, children are creatures of habit. They hate strange toilets. If they are used to the toilet, the two- and three-year-olds find it very difficult to oblige in bed, so it's better to carry them to the toilet and keep to the usual routine. So you see it isn't bed for the sake of bed: It's rest, warmth, and happiness in the most commonsense way. A good compromise is not allowing the child to get fully dressed until officially permitted up. Pajamas, bathrobe, warm socks and slippers should suffice. Then, at least, the child knows not to go out to greet the postman.

Convalescence

Once you get over the high fever stage, the sooner you restore the household to something like normal routine the better, particularly if you have a long convalescence ahead, as for rheumatic fever or kidney trouble. You now have to plan how to fit the child into the routine. There are lots of odd jobs that can be done in the child's room, and it is so much easier to create a calm, peaceful atmosphere in which everyone is confident of the child's rapid recovery if the normal routine prevails. Don't anxiously ask how the child feels. Worry and fuss never cured anybody of anything. The child will be very conscious of your anxiety. Just be interested in all Johnny has to say, plan for his recovery, admire his handiwork. If he's a two- or three-year-old you will have to read and play with him a lot, but if older, will be happy for hours with scissors, a few old magazines, comic books, colored pencils and perhaps a scrapbook and paste, a jigsaw puzzle, construction set, and storybooks. Two good-sized trays will be very useful and save a lot of mess. One can hold a jigsaw puzzle or a card game and the other toys and books. Don't forget radio and television—"Sesame Street," "Mr. Rogers," "Captain Kangaroo," and other children's programs. I wonder what mothers did before TV!

Keeping the child occupied is not the problem it used to be now that we have TV, but don't rely on that too much; it is better for the child to be doing something. There are excellent suggestions in *What To Do When There's Noth-*

ing To Do by Elizabeth Gregg and the Boston Children's Medical Center Staff. This time is also precious in another way! We seem to have very little time to *talk* with our children these days. Life is such a rush, both for us and them, and the generation gap seems to be growing wider. These times when a child is ill are among the few occasions when the mother and child can talk; you will be surprised at how far a conversation can wander from Cinderella along such intricate paths as sibling rivalry, divorce, falling in love, and even ending up in elementary sex education for five-year-olds—all in such a leisurely, natural fashion that there is no tension or embarrassment and youth can begin to learn about life in the best possible way. The same can happen with homework; it is not difficult to arrange for homework to be sent home to the child who has to have a week or so away from school. It would be very upsetting to go back to school and find the class doing completely new work. Keeping the child up-to-date is interesting and not at all time-consuming; in fact, you may wonder whatever they take all day to do at school, and you will build a bridge that you and your child will often cross in the future to explore new fields of knowledge. Many mothers never learn to talk to their children about books and music and everyday events. They are so busy keeping them clean and feeding them and seeing that their clothes are in order that they don't get to know them as people. You can do this when they are convalescing. During convalescence children tend to be emotional, cranky, easily upset, and persnickety about food, so try to be patient and matter-of-fact, loving and kind, even though you feel the opposite. Scolding and punishing do no good at all. Meals are very exasperating. The child is beginning to feel hungry, but is very easily put off and digestion is not back to normal. The child will only eat food that is preferred and only small quantities of that; if jello is a favorite, then you are in luck because you can set fruit in it and make flummery by beating evaporated milk into it. Most children like ice cream and stewed fruit; milk shakes and fruit juice ice blocks can be made at home quite easily. Meat and vegetables are usually the last food they want back, but ask the child, who may feel like chicken in white sauce, or a boiled egg, or even mashed potatoes and gravy. At this stage it is usually a good idea to give a few vitamins, and the doctor may suggest an iron supplement, since infections do cause anemia and affect the appetite.

I think convalescence is particularly boring for the children who must have their activity restricted because of a complication that may not happen. They feel well and it annoys them to be cooped up. Mumps and scarlet fever are liable to late complications. In mumps another gland, such as the sex glands, or the pancreas, *i.e.*, sweetbread gland, may get infected after about ten days; and in scarlet fever a kidney infection has to be watched for after the second week, so the child has to be kept quiet. Chicken pox is irritating; the rash gets itchy and sometimes gets infected. It is better not to wash much, but baking soda in water is soothing and calomine lotion helps. If the sores get red areas around them, however, get an ointment from the doctor.

Children have an extraordinary capacity for rapid recovery; one week they look at death's door and the next week they are ravenously hungry and drive the adults crazy with their energy. If recovery is not fairly quick after the child's temperature has been down for a few days, watch carefully, for there may be an ear complication. Don't ignore pains in the joints, swollen glands, earache, vague stomach pains. Report them to your doctor. And don't push the child too much. After an illness it may be hard to catch up at school. The child may develop some old behavior difficulties such as bed-wetting or stammering as a result of the strain. See that the child gets to bed early, has easily digested food, and not too much excitement for a week or so.

In general, make life as easy as you can and let the everyday world get the child back gradually. Then look back over what you have learned from that illness. If by any chance you had an awful fright because you had neglected to have the child's immunization done, and the doctor suspected diphtheria, don't get caught again. Ask your doctor to see about the immunization against diphtheria and tetanus as soon as the child is fit.

Make sure that immunization against polio has been completed. If the child has not had measles, there is now reliable immunization available. I think it is worthwhile even if it does give the child a fever; at least it avoids the unpleasant complications of measles that are really quite common. Anyway, talk it over with your doctor.

7
The Infectious Fevers

These days the most usual illness accompanied by a fever, is caused by a virus, whether it be a twenty-four hour virus or the kind that lasts months or keeps recurring. You probably wonder if there really are such wretched things as viruses or whether they are another name for diseases the doctor doesn't recognize. Actually, viruses have always been with us. Even pictures from ancient Egypt show the typical paralysis of polio. Then there are measles (German and ordinary), mumps, chicken pox, and the common cold (not the allergic cold). Sooner or later every mother will become familiar with the spots, but the first departure from normal is a fever. First, it is useful to be able to tell that the child really is hot, and a thermometer is a very useful instrument as long as you don't let it rule your life. There is no need for panic just because a child has a fever of, perhaps, 104 °F (40 °C) and is getting near delirium or convulsion level and requires a little sponging to reduce the fever a degree or so. A rise in temperature in itself is a good reaction to infection. By the way, it does not always mean infection; allergic reactions can also be associated with a rise in body temperature.

Many parents have the idea that when a doctor comes he should order something to get the fever down at once, but this is not necessarily desirable, and he may well not be able to make a diagnosis at the first visit. Fever is the first sign and it may be days before the telltale spots reveal themselves; four long worrying days for measles. But German measles, chicken pox, and scarlet fever usually appear on the second. Most colds and sore throats are not going to be serious so don't criticize your doctor if he wisely decides to reserve the antibiotics until he is sure they are needed. It is tragic to see critically ill children allergic to life-saving drugs because they have been used too freely when paracetamol or aspirin would have been enough.

Chicken pox: Chicken pox is very common and very infectious, so you can reconcile yourself to it going through the family, probably at two-week intervals. You may as well let them all come in contact with the first case with some exceptions. Keep grandmother away as she may catch shingles, which is very unpleasant and caused by the same virus; also, if there is a baby under twelve months and the mother has not had chicken pox, which gives the baby six months' immunity, then keep the baby away; perhaps it is just as well to try to stop the father catching it if he has not had it—after all, he is the breadwinner. Unfortunately, there is no immunization yet, and the gamma globulin that can be given to prevent measles after contact does not usually work for chicken pox. The complications are rare, though the rash may become infected with other organisms causing very nasty sores, and there is a very severe type of pneumonia that seems more liable to occur in babies and smokers and people on cortisone.

The rash appears first on the body, then on the limbs and face, as red spots that become blisters, fill with pus, and then scab over and get itchy. The spots appear in batches over several days' time and the child should be regarded as infectious for at least a week after the last spot appears and possibly until the scabs come off.

Baking soda in water, calomine or antihistamine ointment will help relieve the itch. It is better not to worry about a bath until the child is convalescent, but if you do, then use an antiseptic ointment and be careful not to break the blisters.

Measles (ordinary): This is an unpleasant infection with the likelihood of complications. Now that immunization is available, it is worthwhile to get it.

The incubation period is ten to fifteen days, and the child may be off-color and feverish for several days before the temperature really goes up. At this stage the child has sore eyes, probably a sore throat, and appears to have a cold, perhaps with huskiness and a cough. There will be no rash until the fourth day, but there may be little bluish pin-point spots inside the cheeks. The rash is raised red and spreads rapidly, and it appears first behind the ears and on the face, then spreads over the body; it fades in a couple of days and may flake off.

The complications are bronchitis, pneumonia, ear and eye infections and encephalitis (inflammation of the brain), so keep the child in bed and take it seriously until the temperature is normal. It is usual to give penicillin if the child looks sick or has a complication. With measles the fever may be very high and sponging is often needed.

The child is infectious until the rash is gone, and the doctor should see the patient even if you have nursed three others through it already.

German Measles: This is a very mild infection. Children do not seem to get complications, though some of the adults have swollen joints and feel quite miserable.

The incubation period is ten to fifteen days, and though it is better to let children get over it, pregnant women in the first four months should be kept away, and if they are exposed, have protective serum because of the risk to the baby. Children often appear quite well and have a transitory red rash, but some have a sore throat; few will need to stay in bed. A typical feature of German measles is that all the glands in the neck, under the arms and in the groin become enlarged.

Mumps: Mumps is a viral infection of the glands that produce saliva, and the ones usually infected most are the parotid glands, which lie in front of and below the ear; the others are under the chin and bottom jaw. Mumps usually start on one side so that the first thing you notice is a swollen face; a couple of days later up comes the other side. The child may be feverish and very miserable with a painful jaw that can't be opened to eat with. Or he may have remarkably little inconvenience. The kindergartener is rarely very sick, but teenagers can be and are more liable to complications, while adults can really be put out of action. The incubation period is up to three weeks, so this can take some time to work through the family.

There are unpleasant complications such as inflammation of the testes and ovaries causing pain and swelling, inflammation of the pancreas (sweetbread gland) causing severe abdominal pain, and encephalitis causing headache.

The patient should stay in bed while there is any swelling of the parotid or other glands, *i.e.*, about ten days, but complications in young children are rare, so if the child seems well don't be too fussy. Otherwise, follow the general rules of patient care. The diet must be very bland, not consist even of any fruit juice, as this stimulates the salivary glands to produce saliva with agonizing results.

With adults and adolescents permanent damage can be done in some cases if the sex glands are inflamed, but nature provided us with two and it is very rare that both are affected, girls less frequently than boys.

Scarlatina (Scarlet Fever): These days we do not hear much of this infection; it is more often called streptococcal rash, which it really is. The streptococcus causes a throat infection with a high fever, vomiting, and a headache, followed by a bright red rash on the second day. This rash does not appear on the face and is not so raised and mottled as measles. The throat is very red and earache is frequent. In the prepenicillin days, the streptococcus was the main cause of mastoid infections. Any throat infection suspected of being streptococcal is now promptly treated with penicillin and this has greatly reduced the complications, though occasionally kidney infection (nephritis) or rheumatic fever may follow three weeks later. Rheumatic fever used to be a recurring condition that caused serious heart disease, and though this can still happen in the first attack, it is now usual to give long-term pencillin until the child is grown up. Streptococcal infections are very infectious for a week and the incubation period may also be up to a week.

Tonsillitis: The tonsils are two lymphoid glands situated like guards on either side of the pharynx (cavity at back of throat), and this is exactly what they are; they fight off infection and have some part in producing antibodies at least in the first five years of life. Consequently, doctors like to keep them intact. It is only after they have lost many battles and developed internal problems that they are removed.

Tonsils, then, can be infected by viruses and bacteria, and the most serious and infectious are the streptococcal ones mentioned above.

The first sign is usually a fever with a sore throat, If you look down the throat you will see the two red sentinels standing out on each side, almost meeting in the middle at times, and you will feel swollen glands below the angle of the jaw as these are the second line of defense. If the child has adenoids of any size (lymphoid tissue down behind the nose) these are usually infected too, and cause a running nose and pain. The treatment is according to the general rules—bed rest, mild diet (mainly liquid). The doctor must see the child in case penicillin is needed or ear infection is present.

8
The Medicine Cupboard

Every household must have its medicine cupboard, but a very variable quantity it is. No two books or doctors will ever agree as to what should be in it and certainly there are no two identical medicine cupboards in the whole country. For country dwellers it is a more pressing problem than for city dwellers, who can usually dash around to the drugstore, but even hours there are restricted now, so you must all take this problem more seriously. Let us have a look at your cupboard. We will probably have to pause a few minutes while you collect together the things that somehow got into the kitchen cupboard with the food, and the odd ointments, nose drops, and what-have-you scattered around various people's dressing tables. There will still be some things on the list that you know you have somewhere. But let us examine what we have.

I am very much afraid that there are several mysterious bottles labeled, "Take three times a day after meals." Does that "J" stand for John or Janet? You probably will not be able to remember why they were originally ordered, and you will have an uncomfortable feeling that at least one may have changed color since last you looked at it. There is probably a pot of ointment and some pills of doubtful origin.

But let's get to business. First of all, you don't want all those old mixtures. Throw them out, empty them down the toilet; don't let anyone get them! Most made-up prescriptions don't keep very well anyway, but if you have got a few mixtures that you do need to keep, such as asthma mixtures or indigestion tablets, then do see that they are clearly labeled and show what they are used for. Tablets, ointments and powders keep well, but it would be better to throw them out, since the list I have is quite big and needs a lot of room. Perhaps, if you tidy the cupboard and re-label the items, you can keep them. First, for the cuts and sores: bandages, cottonwool, clean white material, a reel of adhesive tape, scissors to cut it or a box of adhesive dressings, a large sewing needle and fine forceps for those numerous splinters you will have to remove, and a thermometer.

If you live in the country you should also have what you need for snake and spider bites, *i.e.*, a tourniquet of broad rubber tubing and some clean cloth or cotton wool to wipe or preferably wash the area as most snakes spill more poison than they inject. There is also a greater chance that you will have to deal with accidents without first aid help in the country, so many people keep good long bandages, slings and something for splints, but I think a rolled up newspaper is as good a splint as any, so perhaps you can leave them out.

You need some antiseptic, though soap and water is excellent for abrasions and cuts; running water hurts less. Most people have their favorite antiseptic, such as Merthiolate or Metaphen, but good old, weak tincture of iodine is still very effective, though it stings. Hydrogen peroxide is very useful for cleaning dirty cuts and removing the bloodstains. Methylated spirits is also a good antiseptic for sterilizing the needle and forceps. Then you need something to relieve pain. The usual pain relievers are aspirin and paracetomol, but most people also keep a combination tablet or powder containing codeine or caffeine, but not phenacetin, which causes kidney damage.

Most people, too, have their favorite laxative for the bowels, but I would like to suggest milk of magnesia for babies, prune juice for children, and a senna preparation or some other vegetable laxative for adults. Certainly no Calomel and no castor oil, unless you want castor oil for dislodging insects in ears, but olive oil is just as good. Paraffin is too feeble for most purposes and interferes with absorption of some foods. If used regularly, add a fecal softener such as Coloxyl. For mild diarrhea of the teething and nervous child I think it is a good thing to keep a bismuth preparation or Kaomagna or some other such mild substance for slowing things up.

I suppose you all treat your own minor coughs or colds when you have no raised temperature, but what about something to clear the nose such as menthol or eucalyptus to inhale, and perhaps a soothing cough syrup, remembering what I said before, to be used only for irritating coughs to allow you to sleep and anyway better bought fresh and no nose drops unless ordered by the doctor.

A few skin ointments will be necessary. For burns a greasy ointment or just vaseline on gauze, unless the burn looks serious enough for the doctor; then you just wrap it in a wet cloth and get off to him as quickly as possible. Sunburn cream is useful for the minor burns and also for sunburn, of course, and there are many good ones available now. For insect bites it would be a good idea to get one of the antihistamine creams, but perhaps it would be wise to keep some insect repellent in the cupboard as well, since prevention is better than cure. And keep an antiseptic ointment for those odd sores and infected cuts.

Calomine lotion and some baking soda for the itchy rashes, Lanoline and vaseline complete my list. No life-saving drugs on it, I am afraid, since they should only be used under medical supervision, and if your doctor is prepared to let you use them in special cases in the country, then you could discuss it with him. For sore eyes and foreign bodies in the eyes, I can only suggest blowing your nose and washing the eyes with salt water—one teaspoon of salt to the pint. I have not even suggested any sleeping tablets, or sedatives, because these, too, should be used under medical supervision. Last, but not least, keep your medicines in a cupboard with a child-proof catch.

You must at times be impressed by the array on the druggist's shelf; there seems to be a cure for everything. Do not be tempted; the less you know about the contents of the shelves, the healthier and the happier you will be. Let your doctor order your medicine when it is necessary, and you are much less likely to take medicine for something you have not got.

9
Vomiting, Diarrhea, and Constipation

In our very hygienic society, vomiting and diarrhea are very upsetting—messy, smelly, and swarming with germs, or so we think as we sit in front of our TV sets watching dying beasties squirming in the drain as Sinko is poured down, or hearing the subtle dangers that lurk in the bathroom and toilet if we do not deodorize and sterilize with Germo. Naturally a modern mother looks with horror at an offensive green bowel movement, and four or five a day with all those diapers to wash can soon reduce her to a nervous wreck. Vomiting is somehow not quite so unhygienic, but it does make the mother and vomiting baby somewhat social outcasts and calls forth much unsought advice from friends and relatives.

Gastroenteritis

The acute summer diarrhea, gastroenteritis, that used to kill many babies is now almost a thing of the past. Better sanitation, pasteurized milk, a war on flies, and better general awareness of the elements of hygiene have greatly reduced this infectious disease, which was mainly caused by bacteria of the dysentery and typhoid family. We still see outbreaks occasionally, particularly in day nurseries and kindergartens, but more often gastroenteritis is a viral infection occurring usually in the winter and is much less lethal to babies. Vomiting and diarrhea cause the child to lose fluids and minerals very quickly, and the vomiting makes it difficult to give medicine. It is horrifying to see how quickly the child can lose weight and the skin become loose, the tongue dry, and eyes sunken, all from loss of fluid. There are certainly times when you need to call a doctor promptly. Admission to the hospital may be necessary to replace the fluids and minerals by intravenous feeding.

When vomiting and diarrhea occur together they are usually due to irritation of the gastrointestinal tract, *i.e.*, the stomach and intestines, usually by infection but quite often by dietetic indiscretions, food poisoning, or allergy. The movement in gastroenteritis is usually offensive, containing mucus and perhaps streaked with blood; it is loose and frequent, perhaps a dozen or more discharges during the day; in allergic and dietetic problems the bowel movements rarely contain blood and are not so offensive or so explosive, but all these conditions can be associated with quite severe tummy pains and a lot of wind. I think that the sudden onset of fever and vomiting closely followed by diarrhea must be regarded as gastroenteritis or acute food poisoning from contaminated rather than indigestible food. Usually, a doctor should see a child with sudden vomiting and diarrhea. The child may be sicker than you think and in urgent need of extra fluid. There is also medication that can help. Antibiotics and sulfa drugs used to be the standard treatment, but viral infections do not respond to antibiotics and these substances may aggravate the diarrhea. It is now considered to be wiser to rely on replacing the fluids and lost minerals and resting the bowel at least while waiting for the report from the pathologist on the culture of the feces. Kaolin preparations such as Kao-magma may not decrease the fluid loss or reduce the fever, but they do make the movement firmer, less messy, and easier to cope with, a fact that mothers and patients appreciate. There is medication that relieves pain and spasm but the morphine preparations so popular in the past are now taboo as they are addictive.

First day diet

An acutely inflamed bowel needs rest, yet since the body must be supplied with water, sugar, and salt, diet is a very important part of the treatment. If the child cannot retain and absorb the fluids, admission to a hospital may be necessary in order to give intravenous feeding as a lifesaving measure. A good indication to the mother of whether enough fluid has been given is whether the child is passing urine. If the urine becomes very yellow and scanty, and the child goes for hours without passing any urine, then dehydration may be setting in. For the first day stop all milk and other food except breast milk and keep to clear fluids. It is rare for breast-fed babies to get gastroenteritis as breast milk contains protective substances, but if they do, they usually are kept on the breast milk with extra water between feeds. The doctor may prefer you to use a ready-made preparation containing sugar and minerals in the correct balance that will dissolve in water. If not, a reasonable procedure would be to use a sugar solution of five teaspoons to a pint of water with some ice cubes and a little simple syrup for the first few hours at least, and perhaps later add a quarter of a teaspoon of salt to the same quantity. But be careful, as too much salt is likely to make the vomiting worse, and when absorbed can be dangerous. Most children do not like these concoctions and will do quite well with water, flat lemonade or ginger ale, clear soups, strained fruit juice or jelly. Whey is quite often recommended in the acute stage. This is made by first making junket, then breaking it up and straining it through muslin, the whey being the strained-off liquid. It is rather a nuisance to prepare, but it has the advantage that it contains some soluble protein, minerals, and milk sugar without the indigestible curd and is well tolerated.

Second day diet

The second day, if the movements are less frequent and the child more comfortable and getting hungry, you may advance the diet a little but still keep it milk free. A reasonable selection would be apple, grated, raw, or stewed, dry toast with cracker biscuits, mashed ripe bananas, nonfat potato chips, fruit juice, and perhaps tea with very little milk.

The third day

The third day may be regarded as convalescence, but still exercise great caution with food or it may start over; rice is a good bland substance either as cooked rice or rice cereal, sago boiled with water flavored with fruit juice and sugar or syrup; weak skimmed milk or 1 in 10 condensed milk may be used on the rice cereal or on well-cooked rolled oats, apple, paw paw, banana, fruit juices, jellies. You may progress gradually to lean meat, coddled egg, cornflour, puddings, mashed potato and pumpkin, steamed fish, and soups.

As the movements become better formed you increase the food, introducing milk very gradually and leaving whole grain cereals and green vegetables to last. It is best to be cautious with fats for a while and certainly keep away from fried food until the movements are back to normal; a scrape of butter or vegetable oil on toast or biscuits is quite all right, but the cooked fats are to be avoided. Milk may have to be omitted for some time and even be diluted or boiled for weeks as the bowel lining may be damaged and take some time to recover its ability to produce enzymes that digest the sugars, such as lactose of milk and sugar in cane sugar. The teething infant who gets the intestinal hurry-up with every tooth may hardly get back to normal diet and normal movements before the sensitive bowel, upset by previous infection, again hurries food through. When this happens go back a stage in the diet, stop milk and roughage such as food skins, excessive fiber, and bulky greens such as cabbage and spinach; mash the food and keep some Kaolin preparation in the house; of course refer to the doctor again if the child has a fever, is passing bloodstained movements or if they are offensive (maybe all bowel movements are offensive, but if you know as soon as you enter the room that the child has passed a movement then that is more offensive than normal).

Gastroenteritis is infectious, so it is necessary to isolate the patient from the rest of the family, keep the linen, crockery, and toys away from the others, and preferably keep the child away from the communal toilet and bathroom. If it must be used, wipe the toilet seat with disinfectant and make sure the child washes hands afterwards, using a towel that will be used by no one else.

When loose bowel movements continue, it is necessary to have some pathology tests done, particularly if the child is not thriving. For this a freshly passed specimen of feces is put into a sterile container (usually provided by the pathologist). This is examined under the microscope for common parasites, Giardia lamblia, eggs of worms, undigested food, and fat globules. It is then cultured to see if there is a particular germ causing the infection. This will not show up viruses unless special tests have been requested, and generally they take too long to be of much use to the patient. If there is a malabsorption condition present, with the child not gaining weight satisfactorily and having poor muscle tone, then some further tests may be necessary to distinguish between coeliac disease, cystic fibrosis, and lactose intolerance. In allergic families milk and wheat allergy may only be diagnosed by leaving them out of the diet for a time, and it is worth keeping a food diary for a few weeks to detect other foods that can cause trouble, such as tomatoes.

It is usual to give the child with loose bowels that go on for longer than the acute attack a vitamin preparation, particularly one in the vitamin B group. If the child is gaining weight and obviously not in pain, then probably this will all pass when the teeth finally emerge, but toilet training will be impossible so that you may have to reconcile yourself to diapers for a while.

Constipation

Bowel problems in children are very common. These days they frequently do not receive sufficient attention. In the past the weekly opening medicine was just about a routine for many families. That dealt with the problem by a good cleanout once a week, and many parents, remembering those days, refuse to subject their children to the same routine, thank goodness. Often the doctor is apt to say, "Don't worry about bowels, some people only have them open once a week." That is all very well; some may, but most have a daily formed bowel action and feel better for it. And now the experts are saying that many of the bowel problems of western civilization, such as diverticulitis and bowel cancer, are associated with our inadequate bowel function, due mainly to our refined diet.

Normally one gets a sensation of wanting to empty the bowel as the waste material passes into the last few inches of the bowel, stimulating the anorectal reflex. The baby simply empties the bowel as soon as this occurs, but during the second year of life learns to hold on. Not indefinitely, however. Occasionally, waiting too long causes unfortunate accidents that often disturb the mother-child relationship considerably. The mother sets the child on the toilet at the time normally associated with a bowel movement but nothing happens. Then as soon as she takes the child off, something certainly does happen, and that distresses everyone. Contrary to the mother's assessment of the situation, the child did not do it to annoy her but was simply too busy balancing on the toilet to relax. As soon as the child felt more relaxed the inevitable happened. Gradually, as he recognizes nature's signals, the child learns to tell the mother when is the appropriate time to go, or goes alone.

This is a sensitive reflex. Many things can happen to upset it and result in the child presenting a bowel problem. But let me make it clear just what constipation is. It is having some difficulty in passing motions; for instance, the motion being hard and large and causing pain, or just coming out in little rabbity bits. The term is also used to describe what happens when there is a delay in waste material passing down the bowel, resulting in days being missed. A form of constipation that mothers often miss until it is a real problem is when the child's pants are soiled frequently with little bits, even with loose fecal matter like diarrhea. This happens when a child has been holding back for days and simply overflows, perhaps not even aware that it is happening, since by then the anorectal reflex is so thrown out of action that the sensation of wanting to have the bowel opened has been lost.

Constipation presents a problem at four main ages in children—in babies, when their milk formula is changed; in the second year, when they are learning control; when they start kindergarten and come in contact with shared, often smelly school toilet facilities; and suddenly, at the onset of an infection, when they have been sweating and lost fluid with fever, and there has not been enough fluid in the bowel to keep the movements soft. Constipation with infection is easily dealt with by giving more fluid, and as the child is not eating much anyway, perhaps a mild aperient after two days have been missed.

The breast-fed baby passes soft, mustard-colored stools. Breast milk is very well absorbed, so the baby may miss two, three, or even four days with no discomfort. This does not matter, but I think both mother and child are getting uncomfortable after three days, so extra fluid such as rose hip syrup, orange juice, or even prune juice may help. There are some medical conditions that should be checked: for instance, a very small anal passage that may need dilating, an underactive thyroid, a nervous defect in the bowel such as Hirschsprung's Disease, where a child just cannot pass a bowel movement by himself and always needs a suppository, and also defects such as spina bifida, where nerves of the bowel are not functioning properly.

The artificially fed baby has a movement of firmer con-
sistency. Those on cows' milk and dried milk often form a
very hard movement that the baby strains to pass and
which may cause a little tear in the bowel wall that hurts.
The mother will usually see a streak of blood in the
motion, which is a warning that the motion must be soft-
ened or a fissure may develop. Soon the baby will automat-
ically hold back instead of allowing the bowel to open.
Instead of the anorectal reflex acting to empty the bowel,
the opposite can then happen. A change in the milk feeding giving some extra fluid, a fecal softener, adding malt
sugars to the feeding, or starting some cereal and vegetables, are all possible answers to this problem. The baby
who has a problem with a fissure may also have problems
in the toddler and toilet training stage. It may be easier for
this child to hold on, maybe even deliberately. After all,
the psychiatrists say this is the child's first big production,
something self-made and which gives a certain amount of
satisfaction. The child may well prefer to hold on until the
experience can be enjoyed alone, off in a corner somewhere. Some children even smear the walls with it, as
some mothers have found to their chagrin. The problem
may be aggravated by inappropriate toilet facilities, a
small toilet seat that makes it more difficult, or being
propped up without any support for the feet. It is very hard
to push down while you are holding yourself up. Emotions
such as anger and resentment may upset the reflex and a
scolding for the mess does not help. It is essential that the
mother sees the movement is soft and easy to pass and that
the atmosphere is right. The matter of getting a soft bowel
movement is largely a dietary one. Our Western society,
with its soft white bread made from refined flour, and our
processed cereals, have been found to be the main cause of
this problem. This discovery has revolutioned gastroenter-

ology; a high fiber diet will be most efficacious in correcting the problem. The price of unprocessed bran has risen considerably as a result, but it is still cheaper than medicine, and there are many processed bran cereals that are very palatable and can be added to the baby's cereal. Whole grain bread and biscuits should replace white bread and sweet biscuits; extra fluid, more fruit and vegetables, perhaps some dried fruits such as apricots and prunes, and the problems of the hard bowel movement can be solved for the whole family. The kindergartener holding back at school needs some help. Make sure the child knows where the toilet is and how to attend to it alone. It does mean, though, having breakfast early with a high fiber cereal and plenty of time before school. A sensitive child finds school toilets very off-putting.

Constipation should be almost always a preventable condition and it certainly should not be ignored.

10
Convulsions

Seeing a child in a convulsion is a frightening and heart-rending experience, particularly when the child is your own; it all seems so dramatic and so desperately serious. You feel that you must do something at once to stop it, and I am sure that is the reason for the treatment usually recommended, which is to plunge the child into a bath of warm water. I always wonder how many people manage to get the bath ready before the convulsion stops; anyway, mother has tried frantically to do something for a few minutes, and the warm water will help to lower the child's temperature. Suppose we look calmly at the situation, now while there is not a convulsion in progress, and discuss what the mother could reasonably be expected to know about the emergency.

First of all, the actual convulsion is rarely dangerous to life at the time, and the chances are that whatever you do for this one you are unlikely to alter the eventual outcome. What you should know is what to notice and tell the doctor when you phone him, what to do to prevent another convulsion and what acute dangers to life might possibly occur so that you can relieve them.

Causes

There is often a family history of fits more often occurring in boys; some families seem to have more members who have fevers in childhood; convulsions are more likely to occur in children who have had a complicated birth or who are actually known to have had some nervous system disturbance at birth—possibly even brain damage. In the newborn baby, convulsions may come from direct head injuries from a difficult birth or some interruption of the oxygen supply to the brain, but the two most common causes of convulsions that you are likely to meet are fever in the young child and epilepsy in the older child.

Though most fits between six months and five years of age are febrile fits, that is, fits occurring at the onset of an illness, usually when the body temperature rises above 103°F (39.4°C), there are many other causes. Fever may actually be due to inflammation of the coverings of the brain, as in meningitis, or of the brain itself, encephalitis. They can also be caused by poisoning, brain tumor, brain abscess, tetanus, breath-holding attacks. Convulsions must always be properly investigated unless the cause is obvious. The doctor will then usually send the child to the hospital.

The febrile fit occurring in an acute infection such as tonsillitis or measles usually happens on the first day, rarely later, and it may be your first indication that your child is sick, though a few hours of quiet prior to the onset may have occurred. If this infection is meningitis the child is more likely to have a stiff neck and to have been more lethargic before the fit. Measles and mumps may be complicated by viral encephalitis and the fit come on later in the illness. Some children are more prone to convulse than others at the onset of an illness and they will tend to run true to type; they are liable to start any acute infection with a convulsion if their temperature is high enough, just as another child may always start with vomiting.

What to do

It may be possible to avoid the convulsion; if the feverish child starts to twitch or become delirious, usually seeing strange things floating around the room, then sponge both face and hands with cold water, and apply a cold pack to the neck; this brings down the temperature and stops the fit. Be sure to unwrap the child, as often the warm clothes and bedding are keeping up the temperature. Instead of dashing away to get a mustard bath ready, it is much more useful to watch the child. You must see that breathing is possible. You do this by turning the child's head on one side and holding the bottom jaw forward with your fingers behind the angle of the jaw. If you can force a rolled up handkerchief between the teeth, well and good, as long as the tongue is forward in the way I have described so that the child will be able to breathe through the teeth. Spoons and toothpicks forced between the teeth can be dangerous and damaging to the teeth without helping the child to breathe easier. In young children with feverish convulsions, biting the tongue and blocking the airway is not such a risk as with older epileptics, since a young child's teeth are small and the jaw does not have great strength. The child will become blue if unable to breathe, and then you may have to use more forceful measures to grasp the tongue and pull it forward out of the way. If the child does not start breathing, you may have to do mouth-to-mouth resuscitation. This is done by first making sure there is nothing blocking the airway. Then, with the patient lying face up, you hold the nose closed and breathe hard into the mouth a few times; by then the child is sure to start breathing again. Always notice the child's color, what parts of the body twitch, if the child is really unconscious and passes urine or has bowels open during the fit. Call the doctor as soon as you can, but if you are alone with the child, do not leave until the fit is over. If the doctor cannot come at once it is just as well to give a dose of aspirin to help get the temperature down and ward off another attack. Be sure the child is really conscious before you start giving any medicine or drink; otherwise you will do more harm than good.

Breath-holding attacks

Breath-holding attacks must be distinguished from convulsions, though they can end in a convulsion if the breath is held long enough. Such attacks tend to occur in strong-minded, quick-tempered, willful children, who are sometimes also spoiled and who, out of sheer temper and frustration, hold their breath. The child goes blue and stiff and may lose consciousness. Breathing then restores the child, but occasionally a lack of oxygen may cause a fit. These performances must not be taken lightly. It is important to try to prevent them as far as possible by avoiding scenes that lead to such events and by distracting the child quickly. You could actually stop the attack progressing to a full blown one by using cold water or a cold washcloth on the face. The shock will then make the child take a breath, though it may not be liked. But remember, there is some management problem usually involved in causing these attacks and you should get advice about them.

Investigations

The idea that teething, constipation, and worms cause convulsions is incorrect. They may aggravate the condition and they do need treatment, but they are not the cause. Most convulsions have no aftereffects except that children who have them are subsequently very quiet and may sleep for some time. They also pass urine during the attack. If it is a simple febrile fit, the convulsions will come less frequently as the child gets older and may be avoided completely by anticipating them. However, it may be necessary to have a preventive sedative for a time. Some doctors decide to have some investigations done at the first attack, but sometimes the fit is over by the time a doctor sees the child. The fact that it is a febrile fit may be obvious, so the child may not be sent to the hospital. Certainly after the second fit an electroencephalogram should be ordered (E.E.G. are the mystery letters). This is a simple test that charts the electrical impulses passing across the brain. It somewhat resembles electrocardiograph for taking heart tracings and is quite painless and no more disturbing. So there is nothing to worry about. If the nerve impulses are normal, then usually nothing will be done. If they are abnormal, then an anticonvulsant will be ordered, but it depends on the tracing what anticonvulsant will be used and whether more tests are going to be necessary.

Anticonvulsants are drugs that prevent fits. The two types most commonly used are barbiturates such as Phenobarb and phenytoin (Dilantin). The barbiturates such as Phenobarb and Prominal are quite likely to excite the child and Dilantin may prove to be the best to use; there are quite a few other drugs if these do not do the trick. Valium is the one most used for the acute attack if the fit is not settling. Preventive anticonvulsant medicine will be used for a year and the E.E.G. repeated. If it is then normal and the child has had no fit for a year the drugs may be tapered off but two years' treatment is more usual. Do not stop treatment without the doctor's approval. If the medication seems to be upsetting the child, tell the doctor, but in general, fits can do more harm than the medicine. About 10 percent of children who have febrile convulsions are likely to have fits in later childhood, and some of the children with a normal E.E.G. may also require anticonvulsant medication until they are past the age when their temperature suddenly rises to great heights.

11
Coughs and Croup

When doctors refer to the parts of the body concerned with breathing they use the term respiratory system. It is just a brief way of referring to the lungs, chest, sinuses, nose, and air passages. When there is anything wrong with these parts they protest in various ways. Two of the main ways are ones you should know something about—coughs and croup.

Why is he coughing?

A cough happens when the respiratory system is irritated in some way; the brain has received a message from somewhere in the chest saying, "There is something annoying me, remove it," and the result is a cough. Now it is quite obvious that if the irritating substance is mucus and pus from bronchitis or pneumonia or sinusitis, then we don't want it down in the lungs and we want it coughed up, so it would be quite wrong to try to stop the cough. What the doctor does is give a mixture to loosen it up, but most of the time nature is loosening it up quite well and the cough mixture isn't necessary, so don't think your doctor isn't any good if he doesn't give you a mixture. Sometimes there is not much to come up. Perhaps the voice box or larynx is being irritated, but coughing is making the condition worse; then there are drugs that will stop the cough. Sometimes, too, it is more important to have a sleep than cough up the mucus, in which case a doctor will order a cough sedative at night but not during the day.

So if your child has a cough, don't go to the druggist and ask for something to stop it; find out the reason for the cough. If your child has a cold and is still getting some sinus discharge, or even has bronchitis, see to it that the discharge is removed by coughing. Sometimes making the child lie down with the head lower than the body for ten minutes or so in the morning helps drain out a lot of mucus and saves a lot of coughing during the day. The young child swallows what is coughed up, but that doesn't matter. The important thing is coughing it up. Even that awful little cough that goes on for weeks after a cold is not best treated with a cough mixture but with vitamins such as cod-liver oil emulsion or some other vitamin A and D preparation, and sunlight and perhaps breathing exercises. These aim at clearing the nasal passages and removing mucus from bronchial tubes.

Breathing Exercises

Nose—blow each side separately two or three times, not too forcibly; shrug shoulders several times or swing arms and blow nose again.

Bronchial tubes—tip head downwards lying on pile of pillows or lean over side of bed, *e.g.*, reading book for ten minutes, nose-breathing. Encourage cough to get up phlegm.

Common cold

The commonest respiratory infection is the common cold, and we don't know any more about it or its treatment than we did years ago. In children it should never be ignored since, particularly in babies, it can cause some worrying complications, such as inflamed ears, and it is more likely to cause bronchitis than in the adult. Moreover, babies can't drink if their noses are blocked, and they may be more comfortable if they have nose drops before a feed to clear the nose and the passages that connect the throat to the ears. Nose drops are not nearly so popular as they used to be, so do not use any you happen to have in the house; they do not keep well and they may not be the right ones. I feel sure it helps to do what mother probably told you, and rub the child's chest too. Camphorated oil, or one of those ointments that give off a vapor do help, but may irritate the skin and the nose if used too long, and camphorated oil is poisonous to drink, so be careful the child does not get it.

Bronchitis

Some children seem more prone to get bronchitis than others; some seem to get it when they are teething; others whenever they get a cold. Babies who are artificially fed get more colds than breast-fed ones. Immune globulin A present in breast milk, particularly in the early milk, protects against viral infection and several other bacteria that cause disease, but breast-feeding also helps the baby to breathe normally and develop good breathing habits. Children with vitamin D deficiency and rickets also get bronchitis. Children who get frequent colds and bronchitis are greatly helped by doing breathing exercises and learning to use their noses and chests properly. I don't mean deep breathing; I mean special exercises that need to be taught by a physiotherapist, but it is difficult to get a child to cooperate with these until he is three, and he has to be seen by a doctor first.

If the cold extends down into the larynx (or voice box) the child may get croup, and because the baby has small tubes, this may be very distressing and even serious. With croup the child breathes noisily, inhaling with a crowing noise. The younger the child, the more you will see the chest move. The young chest is soft, and you can see it being drawn in as the child tries to breathe. These signs mean that there is a blockage in the larynx, and if the larynx is blocked completely, then the child can't get air, becomes blue, and very distressed.

Croup

There are several causes of croup. Probably the commonest is allergic croup, often associated with a runny nose with a tendency to recur; then there is the huskiness associated with a cold, probably a mild viral infection; these two you can manage at home; both may be helped by an antihistamine and a steam inhalation; they are rarely serious, but if the breathing is noisy and the child distressed, call the doctor. Two other types of croup due to infection are really serious: Diphtheria used to be common and lethal before immunization, and croup in an unimmunized child must be watched very carefully; the other is an unusual but very sudden and dangerous type of croup that can cause death in a short time. It may be difficult for even an experienced doctor to differentiate between these types of croup, so don't hesitate to call a doctor if your child is having difficulty with breathing and it sounds as if there is a blockage in the throat. If the child looks very sick and is bluish and breathless, it will probably be best to wrap the child warmly and take him to the hospital at once. If the attack is not so severe, that is, the child is pink and the breathing noisy rather than distressed, you should start emergency treatment. In most cases the child will respond well. You must get the child to breathe in a warm, moist atmosphere. The quickest way to do this is to run the hot shower with the doors and windows shut, or boil the kettle. Do remember that steam from a kettle is very hot, so don't have it too close. Warmth and moisture work quickly. You can keep it up by putting a wet towel in front of the radiator or boiling water in a frying pan in the room; you may even rig up a steam tent with a sheet and an umbrella and a kettle, but be sure to watch the child carefully.

Even the mild croup will need several days in bed in a warm, moist atmosphere, and then be very careful for a few days to keep the child out of the cold or it may all flare up again. At night it is always worse, so an adult should sleep near the child or stay awake on guard if the breathing is distressed. Hoarseness and labored breathing that keep on for hours leave no doubt as to the seriousness, and these children must be taken to the hospital where oxygen and life-saving drugs and modern equipment for clearing the airway and moistening the air are available. Also, there is no guarantee that the croup is not diphtheria, even though the child has been immunized; a booster dose may not have been given at the start of the school term, or this may be a particularly serious form of diphtheria, in which serum and penicillin may be life-saving.

If you are nursing croup or bronchitis at home, remember that all this heavy breathing makes the child thirsty and in need of a lot to drink.

Well, I hope I have not been too frightening, but croup is a frightening condition. Though the emergency treatment I have described usually gives relief, you must get a doctor to the child who is bluish, sweating, and breathless. It is a matter of urgency, even if it is 3 A.M.; it is one of the few real emergencies we have in the care of children, so I do feel justified in stressing it.

12
Sneezles,
Wheezles, and Itches

Allergic conditions are almost certainly increasing in incidence. There are a great many children, allergic to various substances, who suffer from colds, croup, colic, asthma, hay fever, hives, eczema, and bilious attacks. The parents of these children have quite a problem on their hands and far too many people willing to advise them, so I hope a little more advice does not add to your confusion.

The allergic person

This is not a simple story. It is not just a matter of finding out what causes sensitivity and then keeping the child away from whatever it is, or having the child desensitized. It is a complex problem involving the whole person. Someone who is allergic is disturbed by things in the environment that do not affect most other people. Such a person is often sensitive to foods, dusts, pollens, plants, germs, weather changes, and emotional upsets. We sneeze and cough in a dusty room, our noses and eyes run, and these are normal protective reflexes that we call into action to get rid of something that is irritating the mucous membrane lining in our nose and bronchial tubes. But the allergic person reacts on much slighter provocation, such as when the lawn is being cut or a westerly wind is blowing, and the allergic person does so with much more style, more mucus, more swelling and irritability. Chemical substances (antibodies) may develop in the blood that react with substances such as milk or egg protein. When these foods are eaten, or even if they touch the skin, the body may protest by vomiting, diarrhea, or an itchy rash. The blood, however, may not always show antibodies; they may be in the tissues or not demonstrable at all. Recent research in immunology has shown us how the body reacts when exposed to foreign "non-you" material. Learning how to control these reactions has made kidney and heart transplants possible. There are drugs and hormones that can suppress the ability of the body to react and throw out the irritating substance. They are not without dangers, however, because they not only suppress the reaction to the irritating substances but they affect the body's ability to react to infection and stress. It does not appear to do any harm to apply some weak strength cortisone ointment to an itchy rash for a few days at a time, but it is a different matter to use cortisone for long periods to control asthma, particularly in children. In some cases it is a risk we must take, but we ask for trouble if we use powerful drugs that affect normal body function before using every possible means to diagnose the precipitating factors and treat the condition with safer drugs.

In all allergies there is a big hereditary factor. These allergic children come from allergic families, and though there is a great deal of argument as to just what is inherited, psychological makeup, type of nervous system, glands or body biochemistry, there is no doubt about the hereditary influence; the next generation may be much more concerned about preventing asthmatics from marrying each other than about interracial and mixed religious marriages. There is also a big psychological factor; some cases of asthma and hay fever only occur when the patient is under emotional strain. The fear of asthma itself can so disturb a family that the attacks are made worse. Other factors that may be concerned are infection and the weather, but we do not know why some cannot tolerate high humidity, yet others wheeze when the wind blows from the west. It can be very difficult to decide how much of the trouble is due to direct allergy and how much to other factors and whether it is not a bit of both.

One thing is quite certain: Allergies are hard to cure. Most people have to learn to live with their allergic tendency and learn how to control it. Much can be done to help and often remove attacks.

All this makes it important that in childhood the problem should be faced matter-of-factly by parents and children. The child must not be treated as abnormal or an invalid. Some people have red hair and sunburn easily, some are short and fat, some have excitable temperaments. Yours gets a wheeze occasionally or has a runny nose when the wind blows from a certain direction. So what. Many adult neurotics can trace the development of their neurotic symptoms to early childhood and a fussing mother who convinced them that they were delicate and different from others. Subconsciously they learned that an "attack" often saved them from something unpleasant, such as punishment or responsibility, so in consequence they did not learn to face reality.

Allergy in babies

Allergy in babies: Allergic signs often show up in the first year of life but are not recognized as such. This may be due in part to the fact that so much attention has been paid to balanced diets, milk mixtures, and psychology of infant feeding that we have forgotten the old saying that "one man's meat is another man's poison." Many a screaming, colicky infant may be having food that cannot be tolerated in comfort. Signs that suggest allergy are vomiting, loose, mucusy bowels, wind, attacks of screaming, and rashes such as itchy lumps, scaly, itchy patches, sudden swellings, blisters, and diaper rashes. Noisy breathing or a stuffy or running nose and the allergic baby may be suspected of always having a "cold" and "cutting teeth" with bronchitis! Most allergic children have sleeping problems, too. They look pale at times and sweat a lot. Some are so unhappy that their mothers become frantic and begin to think they dislike the child. Life may be very different if the child no longer drinks cows' milk or sleeps on a kapok pillow. But it is not usually as simple as that, so let's look at some specific problems.

Skin allergy

Infantile eczema is one of the skin sensitivities. The skin is red and scaly first on the face and behind the ears, often around the diaper area and in the creases under the arms, behind the knees, and at the elbows. It can be wet and weepy and so itchy, particularly at night, that a child may scratch it till it bleeds. The rash is made worse by crying; in fact, anything that makes the child upset and flushed makes the rash more obvious and itchier. The rash usually appears by three months of age and is made worse as new foods are introduced into the diet. Cows' milk, eggs, oranges, tomatoes, and bananas may cause the rash to flare up; later nuts (as in peanut butter) and fish may give trouble. Quite often babies are weaned from the breast because someone has suggested that the mother's milk is making it worse. I have never seen an eczema improved by weaning, but innumerable times I have seen it worsen after weaning. It can be very difficult to find a substitute milk that suits the baby; often it means goats' milk or soya bean milk. It can be well worthwhile getting the mother of the breast-fed infant to stop eating eggs and drinking cows' milk, particularly if she has been allergic to them herself, as substances do go through in the milk. Most babies gradually become used to the foods that cause reactions by having small quantities as they get near one year of age, but it seems best to avoid them in the early stages of development. Many are much more comfortable without substances that have upset them until their two-year-old teeth are through. It is then better to introduce these foods very gradually, one at a time, in a cooked or processed form; e.g., cooked tomatoes, ice cream, and cheddar cheese before milk.

There are now many ointments that are helpful; soothing ones that protect the skin from irritation and steroid ointments will relieve the itch and remove the unsightly rash temporarily, but it will come back at teething time and times of stress. However, most eczemas disappear by two years of age or so, the time when the teeth are through. Then the children generally have lovely skin and are delightful, active, and sensitive.

Hives look like raised red insect bites and are itchy.

Urticaria appears as raised itchy lumps all over the body. It may also occur as a giant hive.

Allergic reactions

Swelling and itchiness are very typical of an allergic reaction. You may have seen a person suddenly develop facial swelling and even become very breathless after eating peanut butter or some other food that causes sensitivity. Occasionally, allergic reactions follow immunization. As long as they are recognized for what they are, the baby may have an antihistamine before the next injection, which could be a smaller dose. There are also a great many other conditions that probably have allergic elements, but often do not get sorted out: the child whose cold "always goes to the chest"; the nose picker whose itchy nose is always being rubbed and who snorts and snuffles until the whole family shouts at him; the child who has adenoids and tonsil trouble when under three; the pale, cranky child with circles under the eyes; the child who has severe bilious attacks that last for hours, even days, and recur at intervals; and the child with stomach aches. Just to make it more puzzling, all the symptoms that I have mentioned in this chapter can be caused by things other than allergies.

A careful history of food taken, bedding, general environment and events, and weather associated with periods of feeling poorly will often give clues as to where the main cause lies. With the help of antiallergic medicines (antihistamines) and often some mild temporary night sedative, the situation may be restored to near normal.

Asthma

Asthma: An acute attack of asthma is something any mother may have to deal with, whether it be her own child or a playmate on a visit, and it can be quite frightening. You will better understand what happens in an attack if you think of our breathing equipment as rather like the system that brings water to your house. Just as water from the main dam passes through a purifying and filtering process, air is warmed and filtered by the nose; it is passed down the windpipe (trachea) into the large bronchial tubes corresponding to the water mains, and then through the small bronchial tubes and into all the lung tissue just as water arrives at all the household taps. Trouble can occur at any stage: The water or air can be contaminated, the filter may go wrong, and the pipes can get blocked, but the body tubes, unlike the water pipes, can protest. The delicate mucous membrane lining the whole breathing apparatus swells, the little glands that produce mucus to catch irritating substances pour it out, and the elastic coat around the bronchial tubes tries to pull them shut to keep the mucus and irritants from penetrating further into the lung. When swelling and mucus secretion happen in the nose (filter), we have something like a cold with sneezing and a blocked and runny nose, and we call the result hay fever or allergic rhinitis; in the larynx (voice box) it is croup, with coughing and crowing and varying difficulty in breathing; in the bigger bronchial tubes it is allergic bronchitis with a lot of coughing and noisy wheeze and rattle of mucus and even a fever, but not so much difficulty in breathing; in the tiny tubes it is asthma, so what really happens in an attack of asthma is that the bronchial tubes react to an irritating environment by swelling, producing mucus, and squeezing shut. It is very difficult to breathe air in or out. The child sits up, hunches the shoulders, and strains to breathe. Breathing is fast and wheezy. The child may look pale or dusky and very frightened in an acute attack. Fear, fuss, and panic increase the spasm and the child's distress; calmness, confidence, and planned action help relax it.

Treatment of asthma

It is rare for an attack to be really serious, so prompt treatment in a relaxed atmosphere plus intelligent anticipation are the secrets of success.

When wheezing begins, you get the child to sit down quietly in a comfortable chair, perhaps with elbows on the table, leaning forward if very tight. Suggest that the child try to breathe with less effort, shoulders down, inhaling slowly through the nose and exhaling with a sigh. Supply a warm drink, and if the child has a dry, irritating cough, a cough syrup or cough candy. If the asthma does not start to ease off, give a dose of the child's usual wheezing medicine, provide warmth, and get out a jigsaw puzzle or turn on the TV while you wait for it to act. In most cases this works, but if your child is one who has severe attacks, especially if they are sudden, your doctor may suggest a bronchodilator spray as a quicker method of giving the drug to relieve spasm or a suppository as a more reliable and longer-acting method. In these days it is rare to need an injection. Though the modern inhalators last longer and have fewer side effects than in the past when they often caused palpitations, they do not last long enough to see a child through an attack. Medication should be given by mouth as well. They also may not act if the child is very mucusy as they cannot get into the bronchial tubes. Children produce more mucus and have less spasm than adults, so it is advisable to give the usual four or six hourly wheezing medication by mouth even if the wheeze is easing off and to keep it going until the wheeze has gone.

Germs may grow in the mucus, causing secondary infectious bronchitis, so if the temperature stays up and the mucus is profuse and yellow, treatment for infection such as antibiotics may be needed. Younger children are more prone to actual infection and this may precipitate an attack, but even so, it may be settled just by the wheezing mixture.

A child cannot go to school in an acute attack or with a fever. If exhausted after wheezing all night, then the child needs a day's rest at home, but don't let the child get the idea of being sick. Homework, at least, can be done. A wheeze starting in the morning usually disappears at school. Take the precaution of seeing to it that a dose of medicine is packed in the schoolbag and that the teacher knows the child does get asthma and where to get you if it does not stop. Now that we have very effective preventive treatment in Sodium Cromoglycate (Cromolyn, or Intal, in Australia) children need to miss very little school. This is a powder that is inhaled three or four times a day with the aid of a neat little gadget called a spinhaler. It acts on the mast cells in the lining of the bronchial tubes and prevents the swelling and mucus formation. Some children can manage on two inhalations a day and some need the spinhaler only during their asthma season. Most three-year-olds can cope with the spinhaler, particularly with a whistle attachment that shows whether they are breathing in effectively. It will not work unless it gets into the bronchial tubes, so it is necessary to have a bronchodilator spray five minutes before it if there is any wheeze, or for the younger child, the usual bronchodilator medicine. There are still some children who do not respond to preventive medication such as cromolyn and bronchodilator medication. These previously had to rely on cortisone-type drugs with their problems of side effects. However, there is new progress every year and there are now steroid sprays that can be inhaled that are not actually absorbed into the bloodstream. These can be very effective medication and safer, too. An attack of asthma must not gain a child privileges that other children do not have. This can be very hard to avoid. Do not imagine that I am unsympathetic; I am the opposite. But the best way you can help is to teach the asthmatic child how to control asthma attacks and accept the fact that they may occur again. The sooner the child learns to recognize the symptoms and do something about them, and the less the child believes himself to be an invalid, the better.

There is a dangerous tendency these days to blame all our troubles, psychological or otherwise, on two things: one's constitutional makeup, which we inherited from some ancestor and can't do anything about, or mishandling by our poor unfortunate parents. *Parents* can't win. After all, they provided the hereditary characteristics and the environment, so young moderns, often helped by the psychiatrist, have a wonderful excuse to blame their parents and do nothing about their problems.

You often hear a mother say, "She is just like granny on her father's side, has an awful temper, and must have her own way." Well, she may be like granny, but you have a few years in hand to do something about it. It is fatuous to say, "He got asthma from his grandfather. He used to have awful attacks every night. Poor little Johnny can't even stroke the cat without his nose running." Poor little Johnny accepts the fact that his attacks are inevitable and he will be like grandpa, and his subconscious realizes that this has certain advantages: Mother will rush to him at the first wheeze. He may even have a course of injections against cats' hair and get as far as having bronchodilator sprays and cortisone without anyone realizing that the family attitude is all wrong, that everyone is terrified and does not know what to do, and they may not even know what usually does cause an attack. He may even be using an unsuspected kapok pillow or have a learning difficulty that is causing severe stress at school. Sometimes a child's asthma may cease at school. It could be the climate, separation from home stress, removal from a chain-smoking mother who fills the house with irritating fumes, or the routine, regular meals, regular exercise, and lack of fuss at the school.

Management of the asthmatic child

The management of the asthmatic child is never simple, but there are a few general rules.

1. Get yourself a sympathetic, interested general practitioner. He may like you to see a specialist to help sort out the precipitating factors such as allergies, educational and psychological problems, infected sinuses, and to plan a program of treatment and prevention. In general, this rarely means skin tests for young children, but they may be useful for older ones. In the teens a course of desensitizing injections may be indicated if the asthma is seasonal, but there are exceptions—every child is an individual.

2. Adopt a positive outlook, accept the fact that attacks will occur, learn to recognize the early symptoms, such as running nose or crankiness, and take this as a sign that the child needs a good night's sleep. Take a look at the environment too, and give either an antihistamine or the wheezing mixture. It is essential to understand the medication used, as prompt treatment produces much better results. There are two

main types of bronchodilators—those related to Adrenalin and those related to caffeine, the Xanthine group. Both open the bronchial tubes by relaxing the muscles around the tubes and reducing the swelling. They may be used together. Adrenalin is very rarely used for asthma these days since there are safer, less stimulating drugs than Adrenalin and its close relative, Isoprenaline. These are Salbutamol, Terbutaline, Orciprenaline; and new ones are constantly appearing. They are available as tablets, liquids, and solutions for atomizers, sprays, and injections. The Xanthine group includes Theophilline and Aminophylline, which are available as injections, tablets, liquids, and suppositories. Make sure your doctor explains their use. A third group includes Cortisones, also available as tablets, injections, or as the new, safer inhalators. Cortisones, however, are still best kept in reserve until all other methods of prevention and treatment have proved inadequate.

3. Start on an improvement in general health program. Look over the child's diet to see that the essentials are provided. See that the child gets enough pleasurable exercise. Swimming is an excellent exercise that helps breathing and is good recreation. See that the child is getting enough restful sleep. Many asthmatics are excitable children with vivid imaginations and they do not seem to need as much sleep as the average person. However, what they have should be peaceful and relatively free of dreams.

4. Make sure you understand the treatment—what the medication is meant to do, and which one to use and when. Have it labelled and dated and review treatment with your doctor at least once a year as new advances in medicine occur. Never struggle on with

frequent wheezing; this can be dangerous. There is always some help available.

The child must learn how to breathe as efficiently as possible. Many have blocked noses and need to get into the habit of blowing them at least morning and night to remove mucus; this tends to drop down the back of the throat causing coughing. They also need to practice nose breathing when they are sitting quietly watching TV. Many get into the habit of hunching their shoulders and breathing only with the upper part of the chest, and others either cannot or will not try to remove the mucus in their bronchial tubes; these can be helped by some exercises from a qualified physiotherapist. But remember, the child cannot do exercises while having asthma and it is unwise to go to breathing exercise classes that are not conducted by qualified physiotherapists. It is, however, an excellent idea to go to a graduated exercise class with a qualified P.T. instructor, such as one that concentrates on general health. They may go into special classes for children who cannot keep up with the rest at first and be graded over into the general class later.

Asthma is a condition that should not be ignored. Children do not "grow out of it"; it does tend to improve spontaneously in the early teens, but the child has a much better chance of reducing attacks if it has been well controlled in childhood and he has adopted a positive attitude to its management, not allowing it to act as excuse for avoiding responsibility. Several years ago there was an increase in deaths from asthma. This was thought to be due to a combination of factors, particularly some of the toxic side effects of the newer, more effective inhalator spray medications, but also people were persisting too long with the sprays before they got expert help. Better understanding of medication, better preventive measures, and safer spray medication have now reduced the death rate, but we must always remember that every child who has had an attack of asthma knows the fear of death and so do his parents; it is terrifying not to be able to breathe. Courage, common sense, and understanding of the problems and the treatment of asthma is essential.

13
Mommy, It Hurts

Of all natures's danger signals, the one that really gives you the red light is pain. No one ignores pain; you may try to, but it is very hard and usually not wise. If you have twisted your ankle and it hurts, then nature is politely informing you that you must support it. Pain does not necessarily mean physical damage, but it does mean attention is required. You may have a headache and nothing wrong with your head, except that you have had a difficult day and the steadily rising nervous tension has caused a spasm of blood vessels and a headache. The pain is just as real as the pain of appendicitis, and it is just as necessary to relieve the tension as it is to remove the appendix.

Adults can recognize many varieties of pain and tell very accurately where the pain is, but children cannot do this very well. They feel pain but cannot express it adequately in language. A baby can only cry; even when twelve months old the child with a sore throat may only refuse to drink or pull away a sore hand or foot and cry; a two-year-old may groan "sore" or "ooh-ah" and hold up the offending foot or point to the mouth, but it is all very vague. A three- or four-year-old may tell you quite emphatically about a headache, but point solemnly to the stomach when asked where the pain is. The child knows a headache is hurtful to mommy or daddy, so decides this pain is a headache too. Often the parents get annoyed and say the child is lying, when actually the child is only trying to describe the sort of pain often heard about.

Interpreting pain in children is not easy. You need to watch them closely and you have to understand their language, even when the form of expression is only crying. If you cannot understand them, then you do what you would do for anyone else whose language you cannot understand: You get someone to interpret, and if it is important enough, you try to learn the language for next time.

Pain in the tummy

One of the commonest pains of childhood is the pain in the tummy and probably 95 percent of these are of little importance, but they still have to be taken seriously. I am sure no doctor will challenge my advice to refrain from giving opening medicine for a pain in the tummy. It is not wise to do so until you are quite sure of the cause, and then never give castor oil. If you still have a bottle of castor oil, then throw it out; it does not do any good and in the 1 percent of serious tummy aches it could be fatal, so why take risks?

Any pain in the intestines can be severe. You are familiar with indigestion, and at some time or other have felt the agonizing pain that we call wind, which is due to distension plus tension and spasm in the wall of the stomach or intestine. You are familiar, too, with the acute pain of a bowel upset, when the bowel is trying to hurry out something that is irritating it and part of the intestine is in spasm. Pain always occurs when the bowel is stretched and is trying to squeeze back, thus causing a rise in tension. This is the sort of pain that happens when a hernia gets stuck.

Hernias occur when the bowel pushes its way through a weak area in the wall of the abdomen. The common areas are the groin, down into the scrotum, and the navel. Hernias through the navel (umbilical hernias, as they are called) tend to recover without operation, but we sometimes strap them over to keep them in and hasten recovery if they are constantly getting pushed out. They never get stuck, and though they may cause colic they do not really cause trouble. Vomiting, pain, and a lump in the groin need urgent attention, but it will usually go back and an operation will not normally be necessary before two years of age.

All pain caused by a rise of tension in the bowel is severe, and I think there is every reason to believe that a baby with wind is having a very bad time indeed. The child will protest mightily, scream, go red in the face, and draw up the knees; nothing seems to bring relief except getting up the wind or relaxing the tight little tummy with a hot water bag, a warm drink, or antispasmodic medicine. The cure is to prevent the wind getting there, and this needs investigation of the food and the way it is being given to the child.

As every mother knows, pains in the tummy are very common in older children too, and the thing mothers always think of is appendicitis. Appendicitis is not common in children, but it does occur sufficiently often for us to watch carefully. The pain comes first around the navel, because the bowel feels it is being irritated, but is vague as to just where, so it gives a general sort of ache as warning.

The pain of gastroenteritis is in the same place; then as all the bowel is irritated, the pain spreads all over the abdomen. In appendicitis, as the inflammation becomes more definite in one spot, the pain often moves over to the right side. Pain is usually the first complaint, but it is usual to feel sick or vomit.

Children often get abdominal pain with tonsillitis, pneumonia, and other infections, so the diagnosis can be very difficult. Probably the trickiest red herring is that awful pain in the tummy that is apt to come on after breakfast in a child who has started a new school, or at about examination time. If you ignore it, it is sure to be something serious, but usually the treatment is not an operation in the hospital, but a little strategic operation planned to make school more attractive, or the mental stress a little less.

If you want a rough, general guide as to what to do when, for example, your little boy complains of a pain in the tummy, perhaps this will do. Tell him to go and lie down, take his temperature, give him a hot-water bag, and nothing to eat except a drink of water if he is thirsty. If he is still on the bed and complaining of pain in two hours, then ring the doctor or take the child to the hospital. Now that is a very rough guide. The pain may be obviously so severe that you call the doctor earlier, or the child may have a fever or look shocked and pale; then, of course, you do not wait. He may just have worms or vague pains and you feel safe in waiting longer; but it is better to err on the side of safety with abdominal pain.

If the bowels are open, look to see if any blood has been passed or if the movement is loose, green, or offensive. If the child wants to pass urine, see that it is passed into a bottle, ask if it hurts, notice the color, and keep the specimen for the doctor. The child may also be quite likely to vomit, so again notice anything abnormal about the vomit: undigested food, blood, or any peculiar smells or objects. Babies under eighteen months are rather a special problem; gastroenteritis can be serious for them, and intussusception, where the bowel becomes blocked, is a very serious condition. Do not take risks with the little ones.

Earache

One of the most severe pains is the sudden, acute pain of middle ear infection. A rise in tension in any organ causes pain, but the middle ear is a very small space and sudden swelling with infection is a common cause of children waking and screaming in the night. The outer canal leading from the eardrum to the surface is also narrow and an abscess in that can be intensely painful. A baby with an earache may only move the head from side to side, pull at the ear in question, and cry. Or the first inkling you may have of an ear infection is that after screaming for some time the baby suddenly stops and you find discharge on the pillow or, when washing the ears, in the ear čanal. If this happens, don't poke in the ear or clean it out, just wipe away the outer discharge and get the doctor to have a look. Discharging ears are always a matter for attention, particularly if the ear has been discharging for a week or more and if it tends to happen again. Deafness may be the result. The treatment for acute inflammation of the middle ear is by antibiotics—usually penicillin for about ten days, and perhaps some ear drops. If the attacks keep on recurring the child may have enlarged adenoids or some allergic reaction in the nose that keeps the whole area swollen and liable to infection. In that case, some regular preventive treatment may be needed. In some cases adenoids, but rarely tonsils, will need to be removed. Occasionally the infection may spread behind the ear to the mastoid area, but these days it is usually treated quickly enough with an antibiotic to prevent that complication. A condition seen quite often is "glue ear." This occurs in young children who have had ear infections that have been treated; yet the child appears to be partially deaf. The deafness is often missed as parents think that the preschooler is just taking no notice and the child himself does not complain; often both ears are affected. If it is only one, the deafness may be missed and only detected through a medical examination, since the child hears well with the other ear. In this condition there is a collection of fluid behind the eardrum, rather sticky stuff with no germs in it, that can just glue up the works if left but which can permanently affect hearing. The treatment is draining the middle ear by making a small hole in the drum and usually inserting a small plastic tube, leaving it there for months. At the same time the doctor may decide to remove the adenoids and put the child on antiallergy medication, such as antihistamine. The results are good but the big problem for the child is that no water must get into the ear until the tube comes out and that can be a big problem in the summer. There are other causes of earache. Many children complain of it when they are teething or have a decayed tooth. Babies just pull their ears; this is referred pain and not as severe as the pain of acute inflammation.

Teething

One pain that is worse at night is the boring ache of bone pain. It is highly probable that as teeth push through bone, babies do get this sort of pain; obviously they do not all get it, but some people feel pain more acutely than others, and certainly some babies do have trouble getting teeth. Do not get too exasperated with the child who bumps shins and plays happily during the day, only to wake up in the night with the pain. It is worse at night, and, besides, everything feels worse at night when it is dark and lonely.

You will often be surprised and annoyed, too, with the child who one minute seems in severe pain and the next has forgotten it. But remember that children are easily distracted and their attention caught by an exciting game. At times they even crack hardy to be allowed to go and play, so we should take notice of their pains. If you insist on rest in bed as treatment, the "put-on" soon gets better and you get a clearer picture of the real one.

> *Sammy said*
> *He'd a pain in his head,*
> *So Mother just took him*
> *And put him to bed....*
>
> *Though Mother has called him*
> *Her sick little lad,*
> *I really don't think*
> *He can be very bad,*
> *For as soon as I brought him*
> *The little black pup,*
> *He said he was well,*
> *And would like to get up!**

---

* "The Illness of Sammy" from *Dorothy Perkins Children's Verse*, by Madeleine Buck.

Pains in joints

Pains in joints often occur in children: some get aching ankles from relaxed ligaments or incorrect walking, if they walk at all in these automobile-conscious days, and disturbed bone growth at adolescence. Some get aching knees from injuries and posture faults which are very common in school children but the pains to note are the ones that flit from joint to joint. These may be rheumatic, particularly if there is rheumatism in the family. There are tests that can confirm this and there is preventive treatment so that rheumatic heart disease is now much less frequent than in the past.

Headache

Headaches are always difficult ones for the mother to make up her mind about. Again, take the child's temperature. Many infections start with a headache and if it hurts to get the child's chin forward on the chest, then get to the doctor without delay. It always used to be said that a headache at under ten years of age had to be taken seriously, but it is not quite true. Poor eyesight and emotional disturbance will cause headaches, even in the young ones, and the very little ones often do not understand what a headache is. In general it is not wise to give a child a pain reliever such as paracetamol in the way one would for an adult headache. The cause must be found.

Pain, whether it is physical or psychological, is very real, but we always have to be on the alert for the little boy who sorrowfully told his friend on the way to school, "I woke up with a sore throat, and a headache, and an awful pain in my tummy, but it didn't work."

14
Mommy, Come Quickly

Accidents are the main cause of death in all children between the ages of one and fourteen years, and they account for one-third of all deaths in childhood. They far exceed infections; polio and meningitis are mere trifles beside them. In fact, pneumonia, tuberculosis, poliomyelitis, cancer, leukemia, gastroenteritis, kidney disease, and heart disease all added together kill fewer children than accidents. Yet this gets strangely little publicity. A blue baby flies to America for an operation that will not cure it and could probably have been done in Australia; an armless girl flies over to get artificial limbs, diphtheria breaks out in a housing settlement, and they all hit the headlines. A toddler walks under his father's car, or eats pills out of his mother's purse, or falls out of a two-story window to his death, and that rates a little two-inch column over near the market report.

Over six hundred children in Australia and ten thousand in America die every year from accidents—beautiful, normal children, most loved and well cared for by their parents! Yet they die and it is not news. Why is it so uninteresting? Simply because "boys will be boys" and "man is born to trouble as the sparks fly upward." This is everyday trouble, and it can happen to you. In fact, it is highly improbable that you will rear a family without having to deal with some quite serious accidents.

You must learn first aid and accident prevention

As a parent you must do something about it, and there are two things you can do. Learn something about accident prevention and something about first aid. The doctor is seldom on the spot just when you want him. It is usually a frantic mother who picks up the child who has fallen from a tree or down the stairs; it is she who has to stop the bleeding or calm a terrified, screaming child who has been burned. It is actually while the child is in the care of the parents that most accidents occur, so it is our responsibility to prevent accidents and teach the child good safety-first habits.

This applies particularly to drowning in home swimming pools; the statistics show that as many as nine out of ten children who drown in domestic swimming pools either live at the house or are visiting the house as friends. They are not just children who wandered in, and this means that adult supervision of all children while swimming is essential; it is so easy for chidren to trip or bump their heads and panic when they fall into the water.

We all find that children get into trouble regardless of our best efforts. We can only do our best and know some common-sense measures to adopt if accidents occur. Please note the common sense. We doctors just as often bemoan the over-enthusiastic first-aider as we do the completely ignorant, but a little knowledge may save your child's life. Do you know how to stop bleeding? Do you know what to do for the apparently drowned or the seriously shocked? Do you know what sort of behavior to expect of toddlers? Then you will save a life, probably your own child's.

Causes of accidents

The main causes of death in children between one and fourteen are burns, scalds, poisoning, drowning, falls, and traffic accidents. Fatal burns and scalds have decreased because open fires and kerosene lamps are less common. Also, the treatment of burns has much improved, so that children live now who would have died even a year ago. But firecrackers get bigger and better: Empire Day in Australia, the Fourth of July in the United States, and Guy Fawkes Day in Britain always produce a crop of hospital admissions. There are more inflammable fluids than there used to be, and three- and four-year-olds are as fascinated by fire as ever, and by matches.

One to four is a tender age, easily shocked and much more seriously hurt by small burns than older children, so burns still stand as the second commonest cause of death between one and four. This age group has to be protected, but it is a very enterprising and curious age group. Parents not only have to put away dangerous things but have a great responsibility to teach the child a healthy respect for heat and electricity at a very early age. We should train ourselves to put matches away and only to have one or two boxes in use, so that we know if one has disappeared.

Some suggestions for prevention of burns

We can do a sort of "stove drill": firm, flat-bottomed saucepans that do not tip over easily, handles and spouts away from the front of the stove, and no toddlers near the stove. We can be careful about the kitchen floor, so that we will not trip or slip carrying hot liquids. Toddlers so often pull boiling liquids on themselves or get in mother's way and these are terrible accidents: disfigured faces, blindness, shock so severe that a child can die simply from a burned face. So keep the tots away when you are cooking: better screaming in a playpen than crawling around the stove.

We can teach the child, too. A fifteen-month-old infant can learn the meaning of *hot*. I am horrified at the suggestion of some doctors that the parents should deliberately give the child a small burn, for the reaction will undoubtedly be that the most loved person on earth has deliberately caused pain. However, I am entirely in favor of letting the child, in the course of explorations under the mother's supervision, touch something hot. Once the oven door or the hot coffee pot has been touched, the child will be on your side as far as keeping away from heat is concerned. It need not be very hot; just hot enough to teach respect.

The same thing applies to matches. You may hide every box in the house and lock the cupboards. Even though the child knows that hot things hurt, fire is still fascinating and every three-year-old is a pyromaniac at heart. By four the average child will have found a box of matches and set something afire, so surely it is better to let the child have a fire in the back yard, burn paper, use up the whole boxful of matches, and even burn fingers—all under your supervision. Then the child will learn that this is something not to be done alone, that it can hurt and be very dangerous, and that it does not have to be done in secret.

Electricity, too, means nothing until the child knows what a shock is, but not a 240-volt one. Father can organize a little battery shock, and the wireless and radiator dangers mean something then. Two is the age for electricity exploration. The sex most interested is male, of course, so watch those boys. There are very ingenious, almost child-proof, socket plugs that are worth investigating, but like the child-proof medicine containers there is always the exceptional child who works at it until a way to conquer it is found. Parental supervision can never be relaxed despite child-proofing the house.

We cannot keep dangers away for long, or the child will go and find out the unpleasant facts of life and get hurt more than if you supervised him, but he needs absolute protection until he is one. At one he has to understand, no, but you get no real cooperation until he has defied you and suffered, so be ready to comfort and repair the damage that you could not prevent.

Don't forget the sun. Sunburn can be very dangerous, particularly in these days when minimum clothing is in vogue. A child's body temperature may rise to serious heights. It is the area of the burn rather than the depth that causes the general effect, so a small child, red all over, can be very ill. Parents often forget that heat waves are reflected off sand and water and it is not good enough to cover a child with a sun umbrella on the beach.

First aid for burns

Remember that it is not the depth of the burn that matters but the extent and the site; a quarter of the body surface usually means death, but one-twentieth can be fatal if the face is involved. Cotton clothing, particularly flannelette, will flare up and envelop a child in a few seconds; so if you let your child wear flannelette, then be sure there are no fires nearby. The actual treatment of burns changes with every new advance in medicine, but the main risks are infection and shock, so your doctor should see all but minor burns in children. Your first aid must be directed at relieving pain, preventing infection, and combatting shock: If the burns are extensive, cover them with clean material to keep off germs and air, wrap the child in a blanket to maintain warmth and get to the hospital as quickly as possible. *Do not* put on butter or carron oil or antiseptics or tannic acid since it only complicates treatment in the hospital. The whole burned area will have to be cleaned and dressed; almost certainly the child will need an anesthetic and a transfusion of blood serum, will get penicillin by injection, and spread on the burned skin. It will be forty-eight hours before the doctor can tell you the prognosis.

If the area is less extensive, call the doctor or still take the child to the hospital. Burns are intensely painful at first, and this is largely due to exposure to air, so cover the burn with clean material, dry or moistened with baking soda in water, until you can get some vaseline gauze or have the burn properly dressed by the doctor. Small burns are better dressed at once with boracic ointment, vaseline gauze, or one of the antibiotic creams for skin use, not containing an antibiotic that is taken by mouth. Do not burst blisters; that enables infection to get in and, once the dressing has been properly done, do not disturb it for a few days.

The pain passes off in the first hour or so, but aspirin may help, and the hurt, shocked child needs rest, warmth, plenty of fluids and a light diet for a few days. A little point to remember in relieving pain is always to elevate the limb that is injured on a pillow or a sling, for it hurts more hanging down. More than any other accident, burns cause shock and delayed aftereffects that need watching, so take even the mild ones seriously in the sense that you see they are properly dressed and the child treated for shock.

Falls and head injuries

I am sure that every mother wonders how she will ever manage to get her children through the hazardous years of childhood, and every mother of sons is quite an authority on falls. If you call the doctor for every fall from a tree or for every bump on the head, you will find it a very expensive business and you will not be popular with the doctor, so let us consider a few points that may help.

First of all, the elementary rule for illness and injury is rest for the injured part. If the child does not use the injured limb, it is not likely to be harmed, so after a bad fall tell the child to keep still until you have examined it for any obvious twists or breaks or bleeding. If there are extensive injuries, do as little as possible. Do not move the child if you are able to get a doctor at once; just use a rug as a cover to maintain body warmth. However, you rarely can get help so quickly, so an extensive knowledge of first aid is advisable. You should know how to move a patient without doing damage, and you should know how to put on simple splints; a rolled newspaper or a long stick tied above and below the deformed bone, after gently straightening it, will stop further injury to the bone. As far as possible you want to get the child into a normal relaxed position without causing pain. Pain in the neck or back may mean damage to the spinal cord, so the patient should be kept lying flat until the doctor comes. All injured patients are shocked and must be kept warm.

Serious accidents are probably not one in a thousand, and what you want to know is what to do with the sprains, twisted knees, cracks on the head, falls on elbows, and cuts that you see every day. Well, the same rules apply really, and you will have much more confidence if you have studied the first aid book or, better still, done a course with the Red Cross Voluntary Aid Detachment.

Make the child rest, elevate the painful part, and apply cold compresses to sprained ankles and bumps on the head; this tends to stop bleeding and keeps down the size of the lump. Bandage a sprained knee or ankle to support it, but be careful not to do it too tightly, particularly if you are using a crepe bandage. There is bound to be more swelling, and you may disturb the circulation. Keep the child from standing. If there is not much bruising or swelling the next day, it is almost certainly not broken, but a torn ligament can be very painful and slow to heal; it will need support and is better seen by the doctor. Children often get what we call green-stick fractures; they are really cracks or bends in young bones that have not broken through. They need the same treatment as more serious breaks, but they heal more quickly. Children are also more likely to injure wrists, knees, and elbows than adults; these are young, growing bones and easily damaged, so that any joint that stays swollen and painful after a day should be seen by a doctor. It is a good idea to be able to put on bandages and slings efficiently and, like resuscitation of the drowned, you simply can't learn without looking at the pictures and practicing, so get the first aid book and spend a few hours with it.

When a child has received a blow or a fall on the head, the important things to watch for are: loss of consciousness, vomiting, and bleeding from the nose or ears. There is often a concussion; that is, bruising of the brain even without a fracture. After any head injury, rest should be provided. The child will almost certainly go to sleep and may vomit once just after the fall. If vomiting occurs a second time, or there is any bleeding or loss of consciousness, the child should be seen by a doctor, who will almost certainly want an X ray. Once sleep comes it is sometimes difficult to tell if the breathing is normal or not. Quiet, rhythmical breathing usually tells you; however, the real test is whether the child can be roused. You can, if in doubt, try a gentle wakening, for the child will soon fall asleep again. The size of the lump does not mean anything, except that a blood vessel has been broken, and this does not matter if the other worrying signs are not there. For several days after a concussion a child may be tired and cranky, so see that rest is enforced.

Some other accidents

There are a few other accidents you should know something about; little children often put things in their ears, mouths, and noses and throw things in each other's eyes. If a child suddenly becomes blue and breathless, the situation is urgent; there may be something in the mouth that has been inhaled into the windpipe or farther down into the lungs. If rapidly upending the child with smacks on the back fails to get the object out, then get to a doctor or a hospital as quickly as you possibly can. If the object gets past the windpipe into the lungs, the urgency may seem to have disappeared, but if the child is still coughing, or if you did not get the object out, then get off to the hospital just the same.

The things that often get into noses and ears are beads, paper, and bits of plants, and the first indication may be just a smelly discharge. In fact, if a child between the age of one and two develops a smelly discharge from one nostril, the chances are something has been put up the nose; any effort on your part will only push it up farther, so go to the doctor. You will be surprised to know how often the doctor extracts paper, beads, or flower petals, all unsuspected by the mother. Beads in ears get stuck in wax and are too easily pushed farther, so leave them to the doctor. You can, however, do something about live insects. They get caught in the wax and and make a terrific noise, but a little lukewarm oil soon subdues them and floats them out.

When dirt gets in an eye, try to prevent the child from rubbing the eye when it is shut. The child should be made to blow, and if that does not dislodge it, gently wash the eye with water or boracic water (one teaspoon to a pint of lukewarm water). This is usually successful, but it may not move anything stuck on the clear part of the eye over the pupil. Never touch this part; you may damage the eye, but you will not do any harm lifting dirt off the inside of the eyelids with a clean handkerchief. If the eye still feels scratchy and cannot stand the light after half an hour, then you had better get expert aid.

Bleeding

Bleeding is one of the emergencies when time is really precious. Many people panic at the mere sight of blood, while others seem to think that just saying, "I can't stand blood," excuses them from doing anything about it. But we mothers cannot afford to be such delicate creatures. We are almost certain to have to deal with this emergency some time, even if it is only a nose bleed. So here are two points for you to think about: To reassure you, the first is that blood makes an awful mess and always looks more than it is; to stir you to action, the second is that bleeding must be controlled as quickly as possible. The younger the child the more serious blood loss is likely to be.

A certain amount of bleeding from a wound is a good thing; it washes out germs, and a stab wound with little bleeding is more prone to infection; in fact, tetanus germs can grow only when they are buried away from air as in an injury sustained with a garden fork. Deep cuts around wrists, ankles, or fingers often mean severed tendons, and should be seen by a doctor as soon as you have controlled the bleeding. Unless there are fragments of glass in the wound, direct pressure at the site of hemorrhage is usually the best treatment. This is done with a piece of clean material, a pad of cotton wool, and a firm bandage. If the blood comes through, do not take off the first bandage; apply another over it. Always remember to raise the bleeding limb; it bleeds more hanging down. It is very seldom that you need to stop the circulation by tying something around the limb, but if you do, the tourniquet shoud be loosened every half-hour and reapplied while you are waiting for help. However, lives have often been saved by someone on the spot at an accident being able to stop the bleeding from a large artery by pressing on the point where it is most easily compressed. Here again, this is not a first aid book, so consult one for the pressure points. Also, remember that it takes three minutes for blood to clot, so do not keep peeping at the wound or dabbing at it. Nature likes five minutes' pressure and she will stop it her way even without pressure, except where arteries and big veins are cut.

Nose bleed

Another hemorrhage you will almost certainly have to deal with is the nose bleed. Nose bleeds are fairly common in children and the reason they occur most often in early spring is probably that this is the time for colds, westerly winds, and the allergic reactions, so the child's nose gets sore and crusty. The child picks the crusts, causes bleeding, and will not leave them alone, so if he breaks into a little net of blood vessels there can be quite brisk bleeding. The best treatment for the actual hemorrhage is to make the child sit up, leaning slightly forward. Hold the child's nose gently but firmly for five minutes by the clock. The aim of cold compresses to the nose and back of the neck or, the old wives' tale, keys down the neck, is to cause blood vessels to constrict and stop bleeding, but direct pressure is most effective.

Once you have stopped the bleeding you must stop the nose-picking, if that was the thing that started it. First moisten the crusts by leaving a wet swab of cotton wool in the nostril for an hour or so, then remove them gently and vaseline the nostrils to stop the crusts reforming. If the child has frequent nose bleeds, a doctor should be consulted. The bleeding usually comes from a damaged blood vessel in the front part of the nose and more active treatment may be needed. The treatment is quite simple for the ear, nose, and throat doctor, and it is foolish to allow the child to get anemic from blood loss.

Everyday cuts and scratches

Just a word about the everyday cuts and scratches. I suppose you all have a favorite antiseptic, but I would like to mention a few points you may not have realized. The first is that soap and water clean a wound best; use a pure soap and cotton wool with plenty of water. Hydrogen peroxide is as good as anything for cleaning a dirty wound; it loosens dried blood and infected material very efficiently, but use it diluted 1 part hydrogen peroxide to 4 parts water. Weak tincture of iodine is a very good antiseptic, but it does sting on open wounds and some skins burn if iodine is bandaged on a wound, so many people prefer one of the antiseptic dyes like Dettol, acriflavine, or mercurochrome. In any case, it is more important to clean the wound than to dab antiseptic all over it.

Snake bites

Snake bites, including the bites of trapdoor and redback spiders, are emergencies and are all treated with a tourniquet. The tourniquet should not be too tight; you want to stop poison getting into the circulation, but if blood can get into the limb the wound may bleed and get rid of the poison. Wipe the bite first to remove poison from the skin. Otherwise do not cut it or you may actually let more poison in. Then get medical attention as soon as you can. The emergency treatment, however, is what saves life.

Dog and rat bites can mean infection with tetanus and possibly need an injection of penicillin. Of course, you should have had the child immunized against tetanus as a baby, but a booster dose is still needed after many injuries.

So much for the emergencies. It is foolish to fear things

that may never happen, but it is never foolish to take commonsense precautions and to prepare yourself to cope with
the everyday possibilities.

What's in the child's mouth

"What is in Johnny's mouth?" Every mother must have
asked that question many times and gasped with relief as
she extracted the offending object just in time. You cannot
possibly anticipate every accident, but you can train yourself to be careful about needles and pins, have a medicine
cupboard and use it, and above all not to carry pills in
handbags. Small, smooth objects such as buttons, beads,
and seeds slip down easily and turn up in a day or so in the
motions. The dangerous things are sharp or irregular
objects, and poisons.

Poisoning

Poisoning is not nearly as common an accident as falling
over or being hit by a car, but under the age of three it is
very serious. Under one, when the child is crawling everywhere, and everything goes in the mouth, poisoning can be
a problem. Little boys particularly seem to find a great
many dangerous things. Little girls seem to get into more
trouble with poisons when they are about three; I suppose
it is because they stay with their mothers and play with
their handbags, while boys tend to get out of doors away
from the household dangers.

The accident surveys show that poisons are usually
either in use or just not put away when the child gets them.
Often it is not necessary to climb to inaccessible places or

force locked doors. They also showed that many parents
did not know the substance they were using was dangerous; in fact, they were often labeled "noninjurious," meaning noninjurious to the kitchen sink or the toilet, not the
baby's insides. So, though many of these parents were very
conscientious people, they were not careful enough simply
because they had not thought about it.

Kerosene

Kerosene is a very common cause of poisoning. It may
be found in every household as fly spray, a cleaning preparation, or for lighting or heating; in the country as
kerosene used for generating power, which is very dangerous. You may even have some household kerosene in a bottle labeled *sherry* or *vinegar*. One tablespoon of power
kerosene can be fatal to a twelve-month-old child if swallowed, but even one teaspoon of household kerosene inhaled into the lungs may cause lung irritation that can kill
or cause pneumonia. For this reason a child who swallows
kerosene should not be made to vomit; better to give a
drink of milk (evaporated for preference) and get to a
doctor.

You see what I mean. It is the everyday things you have
to watch, the disinfectants you so often keep in a very
accessible cupboard under the sink. Lysol and its relatives
are terrible poisons. Most of us are very careful about rat
killer and ant killer and so we should be; they are so sweet
and attractive to children. Also, father is not always so
alert to danger while he is actually using them or the garden insect sprays. It is not just a matter of seeing that they
are put away either; it is that old problem of keeping an
eye on the two-year-old.

Medicines

Three hundred and seventy-four children who took poison in one series managed to sample sixty different poisons among them, with medicines, tonics, and pills of all sorts high on the list. Mother's iron pills, her sedative pills, sleeping tablets or headache pills are often in her handbag or on the dressing table; allergy pills taste nice and are often not thought of as poison; purgative pills, some of which contain belladonna, can be dangerous, as can quinine tablets and tonics containing strychnine. All of these can kill a child who will chew up two or three tablets as if they were lollipops. Aspirin is now the commonest cause of poisoning in children. Though it is not a very poisonous substance compared with most other medication (a twelve-month-old child could eat three tablets without dangerous results), children die from it every year because it is often misused and is easily available. The dose for a three-month-old baby is less than one-quarter of a tablet and if an overdose is repeated several times in the night, as it often is, a baby can become very ill. One of the symptoms of poisoning is also misleading: It is fast, noisy breathing that can be mistaken for breathing difficulty due to a cold, so the mother may make the mistake of giving more aspirin. Most headache pills now contain other things as well, and we need to be careful. Some of these with aspirin cause serious kidney damage. In fact, in Australia the main cause of kidney failure requiring kidney transplant is combination headache tablets, largely consumed by women. Sedatives are now in nearly every home, usually as quite small and attractively colored tablets; sulfa drugs are also in far too many homes and can be dangerous. All cough mixtures, particularly the syrups, which are so nice that the child could drink a bottleful, often contain strong cough sedatives and could be fatal. Calomel is a very dangerous aperient that has now nearly disappeared from the average home. If you still have any, get rid of it.

There are many medicines that are harmless in the dose ordered, but if the baby gets them they are dangerous, so it has been suggested that poison labels should be used more freely to enlighten parents. Many pills are now in foil or sealed plastic wrappers that make them more difficult to get at, but if they are not, make sure they are in a screw top jar, preferably the child-proof variety, and kept in the medicine cabinet, not on the dressing table or in a handbag. In any case, they should all be in the medicine cupboard. Disinfectants and antiseptics are found in every home too, and they are so easily left on the table while we go to the phone.

Disinfectants and insecticides

Carbolic and caustic soda cause horrible burns. Even half a teaspoon of carbolic swallowed by a one-year-old can be fatal, and even less can cause such burns in the throat and mouth that the child dies later. So do be careful, and keep them out of reach. The disinfectant oils commonly used are relatively safe; a tablespoon is necessary to cause serious effects, and since they smell and taste so strong, the child is unlikely to swallow as much as that. Ink and shoe polish may contain poisonous dyes and chemicals, but they are low on the danger list. Matches and their containers are now fairly safe, though I would not recommend them as an article of diet. Plant sprays contain arsenic and nicotine, and rat bane contains arsenic and phosphorus, all deadly poisons. A very common rat poison now used is one that stops the blood clotting so the animal dies by hemorrhaging into its tissues. I have seen children covered with bruises and the parents suspected of child bashing when a child has eaten this kind of rat poison.

Flypapers, if you ever see them now, taste rather nice and contain arsenic. A common poison is nicotine; a few drops of garden nicotine could be fatal; a whole cigarette can make a two-year-old very sick. Fortunately, not many will eat even a cigarette end, but that is still no excuse for the nicotine addicts who throw their butts where there are children. A pet abomination of mine is the woman who feeds a baby as she smokes, or just after a cigarette, and often does not wash her hands. Babies get quite a lot from the mother's fingers.

Other household substances to watch are methylated spirits, brandy, gasoline, and paints that contain lead. Lead is not an acute poison as a rule, though sucking batteries can produce rapid effects; it is a nasty, insidious poison and hard to detect, and children may get it from eating flakes of paint off the wall or licking dewdrops from painted railings as so many did in Queensland years ago, or even sucking lead toys. Lead cannot be washed out of the stomach and got rid of easily; it does permanent harm to organs and inevitably shortens life. There is now considerable concern about the amount of lead being inhaled in gasoline fumes as in one Australian city and in American cities near freeways it has been found that the level of lead excreted in the urine of children was enough to cause harm to brain and blood.

Handle poisons safely

It is certainly the mother's responsibility to train herself to handle poisons safely, putting stoppers and lids back as soon as disinfectants and polishes are used, and keeping the poisons in high cupboards and the medicines locked up, never putting poisonous substances in food containers such as soft drink bottles. But is there anything we can do about educating the child? The dangerous age for poisoning is nine months to three years, a very inquisitive age— into everything, tasting everything, and getting everywhere. They have no judgment, little appreciation of danger, and an amazing capacity for getting into inaccessible places. The younger they are the more promptly things go into their mouths. The older ones are great imitators; they want some of mommy's medicine and some of what daddy has in the bottle. You cannot blame them if they eat pills when they see you having them. So I think we should take our medicine in private; after all, why should a child know all about his parents' medicine? Some experts even suggest that we should put something nasty in a bottle and deliberately leave it about; perhaps it is worth doing for a two-year-old who still puts everything into the mouth and the active, exploring child who is always in trouble. Otherwise I am apt to think it is the mother's responsiblity to keep things away.

What to do if a child takes poison

Investigations into accidents also show that an important point in saving the lives of children was to get prompt treatment.

If you think your child may have taken poison, then get to the nearest hospital without delay; don't wait to see if anything happens. By then it may be too late. The aim in treating poisoning is to remove the poison if possible, and counteract the effect with an antidote and something to delay absorption. Try to make the child vomit, unless kerosene or something that has burned the mouth has been taken, or unless the child is unconscious. In these cases, vomiting is more dangerous than leaving the poison down until the doctor sees the patient. It is usually best to give a drink of milk or even water before pushing your finger down the child's throat. The most effective medication to make a child vomit is Syrup of Ipecac, and this is a useful substance to keep in the medicine cupboard. The recommended dose will usually make a small child vomit fairly soon. However, a very effective way is to put your finger in the child's mouth until you reach the back of the throat, then rub it. This irritates the pharynx and will usually produce vomiting quite quickly. If this does not work, then give some more milk and try again. You may get bitten, but with food in the stomach, the child will vomit eventually and the milk will have delayed absorption. The milk is also soothing to an irritated stomach. When you get to the hospital, the stomach will probably be washed out with a sodium bicarbonate solution through a stomach tube and the child kept for observation. It is important to take with you the empty bottle or whatever you think the child took, plus anything that has been vomited, so that the poison can be more readily identified.

A stomach washout is a nasty experience but much safer than leaving down a possible poisonous substance. Besides, it is not an experience that a child wants to repeat. Caution in the future about tasting those pretty tablets will undoubtedly be the result.

SOME SUGGESTIONS FOR
ACCIDENT PREVENTION

Since your child is going to acquire your attitude toward driving a car, then drive with safety in mind—as if you were giving instruction—for that is what you are actually doing.

No matter how carefully you drive and no matter how well you train your child to drive and manage a car, there will always be dangerous drivers on the road. From baby-hood adopt safety measures in the car.

Teach children to understand and observe the traffic regulations from a very early age. Make a game of it; teach them to notice the breaches of regulations they see pedestrians and other drivers commit, and in this way they become aware of the regulations and the reason for them.

Learn what behavior to expect of children at each age, and above all, learn to appreciate the toddler's insatiable curiosity and inability to foresee danger.

Teach children to respect the common dangers—water, fire and new tastes—and teach them it hurts to fall from high places and that moving objects must be treated with respect.

Your children's safety is your responsibility until old enough to take care of themselves. This means constant vigilance until five, full appreciation of an inadequate sense of responsibility until ten, and continuing awareness of their needs through adolescence.

Never leave children under the age of nine alone in the house.

Learn something of first aid, so that you are a help, not a hindrance, in times of emergency.

Do not nag a child over trifles such as manners, toilet training, and thumb-sucking, and the child will take more notice of your insistence on safety first and will live to acquire good manners.

15
The Special Child

The handicapped child

The child with a physical disability has more to over-come than the actual handicap itself. Being different from others the same age, there are many activities that are off limits; children are not kind to those who cannot conform to the group. The child may easily become angry, resent-ful, and bitter, or completely dependent on the family; some children with a handicap use their disability to avoid difficult tasks and facing up to life. A disability in other children can become a challenge that spurs a child to de-velop strength of character and a degree of achievement far beyond expectations. So much depends on the attitude taken by the parents. It is so easy to overprotect such a child, since one's heart aches at the defeats and longs to prevent the hurts. It is more difficult for the disabled child to obtain those three essentials for mental health: to love, to be loved, and to see oneself as a worthwhile person. The child must find some things to do well and must know the security of being loved for just being unique. It is not easy to discipline a small person who is handicapped and make it understood that the child has a place in society, that it is still necessary to earn. I have seen the most tremendous courage in these children and their parents and a depth of love and unselfishness in these families that gave the whole family a quality of life many families never find. I have also seen the tragedy of the handicapped child break up the family. Fathers, in particular, find it hard to accept a deformed child as theirs. There is still a sense of shame and why-did-this-happen-to-me feeling. The extra work, the hesitation to ask friends to baby-sit, the extra cost, the restriction on movement caused by the disability, all may well prove too much for a less than satisfying marriage and it may well break under the strain. In our nuclear family system, where many families have little contact with grandparents and little community spirit, the family with the handicapped child can be very isolated. If the doctor does not know the facilities available in the community to help, then the services of a social worker may be necessary. No family should bear alone the expense and restrictions of the parents who are lovingly rearing their handicapped child. Fortunately, many self-help groups have now formed in the community. For most of the common problems there is now a group of parents who have the same problem and who share their troubles and will help the others to cope. These can usually be contacted through the telephone book. There are some conditions in which the child's future is threatened even more by the doubt as to length of life. Those caring for a child with cystic fibrosis, thalassemia major, and even hemophilia, do not know how long they will have the child with them. These parents often manage to live in the present from day to day making every day worthwhile. They seem to be able to live each day to the full and are happier and less obsessed with the competitive life of their fellows and more aware of the good and enjoyable things around them that should be enjoyed here and now.

Possibly the most demanding conditions to care for are those in which the child has suffered neurological damage and there is some degree of mental retardation or failure of vital nerves to work, such as those controlling the bowel and bladder. There are many children who have had difficult births or have been very premature; those in which nerve cells have been damaged and they are spastic or have partially paralyzed limbs; and there are an increasing number of children who have spina bifida operations. Spina bifida is a condition in which the spinal cord has not closed over properly and there is a meningocoele—a bulging of nervous tissue and the coverings of the cord through the opening in the spinal cord. These cases can often now be repaired, whereas in the past the condition was hopeless. Now many live to have normal intelligence, but they may have bowel and bladder problems. They may even have to live in a wheelchair because of damage to the nerves supplying their legs. Many surgeons will not operate on the severe conditions if they think there is little chance of normal intelligence or reasonable quality of life, but amazing results have been obtained and the work continues. Children who have suffered lack of oxygen during birth and those who have had meningitis or encephalitis may have brain damage. Some of these have damage to intelligence, others to limb movement, hearing, or vision. This may mean years of remedial teaching, physiotherapy, and speech therapy with all the day-to-day management just that much more difficult than the ordinary child. The Downs Syndrome child (Mongol) has a chromosome abnormality and is always mentally backward to some degree. Such a child is lovable, easy to care for, only too often almost a pet to the household. I have seen too many women devote their lives to such children (even to the extent of neglecting their other children and their husbands) to think that their very retarded child should be reared to adult life in the normal family. The most retarded need special schooling and often institutional care to save them the stress of competition with the normal and also to relieve the family of the tremendous stress of coping with the many problems that go with severe retardation. Most mildly retarded children who can look after themselves and attend normal school in normal classes are better at home in a family, but no family should try to cope with severely affected children or even the mildly affected ones without help. Recently there have been some very encouraging experiments in education of retarded children that suggest they are capable of learning much more than was ever anticipated if special teaching methods are available. Most epileptics can live a normal life with no brain damage or deterioration, but they must have regular medication and they must restrict their activity to avoid situations that could endanger their lives or those of others. This includes activities such as scuba diving or swimming alone. A well-controlled epileptic, however, can drive a car but not an airplane or a train. Fits may cause brain damage themselves, so the continued treatment is vital. The cretin born with deficient secretion will need to take lifelong thyroid hormones but has a reasonable expectation of normal living. Life should not be shortened, though academic ability may be a little below average. Most of the children born with defects in the heart, such as the blue babies, and the hole-in-the-heart babies, will now have some chance of surgical repair of the defect. The results here are improving every day. Some are now operated on soon after birth, but most will be nearer four or five years of age if all is going well. Most of the children who develop rheumatic heart disease can now have surgery later if the valves are failing.

The children with recurrent urinary tract infections, with cystitis or pyelitis, present a problem. They often have a congenital abnormality in the kidneys or the passages leading from the kidneys to the bladder, and they may need some antibacterial medication for many years and an X ray of the kidney system to detect any abnormality that may be corrected by surgery. Hare lip and cleft palate can be so beautifully repaired these days that the scar may be hardly visible. There are difficult times in the early years when feeding is a worry and the baby may be plagued with ear and nose infections but these operations are often done in the first year now, at least the first stages, which reduces many of the problems.

Children with cystic fibrosis are some of the most difficult to care for. They are very prone to chest infections. They need special inhalations to combat this and may often have to sleep in special atmosphere tents. Their digestion of food is seriously impaired by lack of enzymes that can, to a certain extent, be replaced. They cannot tolerate heat as the sweat loses salt. It is essential to have such a child cared for by a doctor in a special clinic who is up-to-date with the new research, and who has a hospital affiliation where the child can be admitted at times for reassessment and stabilization.

The children on special diets seem to have very pressing problems. It is very frustrating to be different where food is concerned. The school snack bar presents intolerable temptations. Parties, visits to other people's homes, in fact all special occasions make it so difficult for the child to be different. Diabetes, phenylketonuria, and hyperactivity all have a special diet as treatment. The diabetics have a fairly wide range and can usually choose their food without being too conspicuous, but they must understand the condition and the importance of testing their urine for sugar and regulating their insulin injections (nearly all diabetic children require insulin by injection). The children with phenylketonuria have a very strict diet with special proprietary food without certain protein in it. The food is not very palatable; yet if they allow the body to absorb too much phenylalanine it will damage their brain cells. These children almost invariably do rebel against the diet at times. Hyperactivity diet omits preservatives, artificial coloring, and foods that contain salicylates. That is not easy in our ready-made-foods society with fizzy drinks offered to every child visitor. There can be a great deal of anger and resentment that in the hyperactive child will precipitate worse behavior. The wheat-free diet of the child with coeliac disease used to be very restrictive, but now there is gluten-free bread, gluten-free canned food, and a wide range of suitable foods, so that even if the child must stay on it until adulthood—or even longer—the diet is as healthy as that of the diabetic. The child will look well, feel good, and live a normal life. It can be very good experience for diabetic or asthmatic or crippled children to go to a camp for children who share their particular disability; they learn a lot about management, they become aware of their own responsibility for their treatment, and learn that the success of its outcome will lie with them. The diabetics learn to give their own injections and become independent. The asthmatics learn how to anticipate an attack and what their medicines are for. It is extremely important that all children with a handicap learn to become as independent as possible.

It is in adolescence that the real rebellion usually comes. Every parent must be aware of the adolescent identity crisis and the agony of being different from one's colleagues.

Adolescents may well refuse to take medicine or to eat a special diet. They need great sympathy and understanding and help to find themselves. It is not easy to face the probability of permanent handicap, but it is amazing how many can face life with courage to overcome the handicap or even turn it to advantage. I know of deaf people who can simply turn off their hearing aid and shut out the world, who are capable of the most enormous concentration and not worried by the constant noise that besets our lives.

Caring for the handicapped

For parents caring for the handicapped child there are several musts.

1. Get treatment for the child early, do not accept defeat, and search for an understanding and sympathetic doctor until you find one.

2. Keep up the treatment, have the child reassessed at least every year as new treatments are continually resulting from research.

3. Help the child early to independence and to understanding of the problem and its treatment so that it will be possible to grow up facing up to life and overcoming the difficulties as they arise.

4. Find interests and activities in which the child can take part and excel and do not allow the members of the family to take on the same activity and do better. For example, if the bent of the child is toward music, then let the other children learn different instruments if they, too, must play something.

5. Conduct yourself as normally as possible, accepting the child as an individual having special needs and inter-

ests that must be met just as they must be met for the rest
of the family.

The hyperactive child

Recently, a medical friend of mine from the U.S.A.
asked me if I ever remembered having a hyperactive child
in my class at school. I thought very hard, and despite a
memory that is now recalling the past with more accuracy
than last week, I could not remember a single child who
fitted the full-blown hyperactive child syndrome. Neither
could she. We could remember very active, destructive,
talkative children who often spent quite a bit of time out
in the corridor during school hours. We could remember
lively, happy clowns who saw no reason for work, but not
the hyperkinetic child—child with poor concentration,
endless movement, and a long story of disrupting every
group joined. Is this, then, something new? A development
of the post–World War II era? Is it the result of change in
child-rearing practices? We speak of the Spock-marked
generation, the generation that was loved and understood
and given enough rope to hang itself with few limits set on
anything. Can it be the result of the purposeless do-your-
own-thing philosophy? Is it because these children were
not recognized in the past, just kept out of the way or
sedated into apathy? Is it because parents are no longer
prepared to give the time and patient, loving care to small
children and there are no grandparents around to substitute for them? Is it because children are simply not getting
the continuity of loving care that is needed for consistent
progress? Is it because so many people now impinge on the
developing child and cause confusion? Or has something
happened to change children and produce a new type of

child? Could it be that the amazing amount of medication that now passes to the developing fetus across the placenta during pregnancy and childbirth in some way is affecting the sensitive, immature enzyme systems in the brain? We know that some drugs very commonly used in childbirth do have a lasting effect on the child; up to twelve months has been demonstrated. We know that the children from heavily sedated labors cry more, but could that have just been the type of labor? Maybe that child could have died or been mentally retarded in a previous generation.

I do not know the answers, but I do know that in twenty-five years of consultant pediatrics the problems have changed. Today I am seeing hyperactive babies and incredibly restless preschoolers with poor concentration who come from families that have already reared normal children well and where the parents are sensible, conscientious people whose major problem by the time I see them is exhaustion. I also know that in my practice these children come in the main from allergic families, and that allergy seems to be increasing. Dr. Feingold* is an allergist and I do not think it is coincidence that he observed that certain foods made some children worse. He says it is not allergy. Before his diet came out I had my own list of foods that upset children and they were all on his list. I think we simply do not know enough yet about the type of allergic reactions that occur; immunologists are describing more each year. It seems to me the answer will emerge as some environmental factor in early development—for example, a combination of medication and diet that particularly affects the families with allergic tendencies. But of course there are many already known causes of behavior disturbances in children, many of which involve overactivity.

*Ben F. Feingold, M.D., *Introduction to Clinical Allergy* (Springfield, Illinois: Charles C. Thomas, 1973).

In the meantime, let us keep the whole picture in mind. Our health depends on our heredity, our environment from conception or even before, and the ability of our parents, ourselves, and society to manipulate the conditions in which we rear children. We must realize that some situations will produce children who are excessively active, such as overstimulation to a normal nervous system, reaction of a defective nervous system, and reaction of an excessively sensitive nervous system to an average environment. I have seen too many cows' milk allergy babies who have screamed their way through the first year of life until their parents were desperate and either whacked them or resorted to psychiatrists who then said they were neurotic and unable to cope. I have also seen too many dyslexic children disrupting the class and failing at school to accept the theory that removing salicylates in the diet will help all hyperactive children.

The unmanageable child

Here, then, are my thoughts on the investigation of the unmanageable child. First look at the specific child and the nature of the nervous system. Is Johnny, for example, genetically an excitable, alert child, conscious of every sound and movement, reacting to everything around him? Is he like any particular relative? Is this an allergic family or one prone to psychological illness? Has he passed the developmental milestones at the usual time, or is he behind in one, such as talking? Does he appear to have a specific difficulty in learning, or does he seem to be generally retarded? Could this child have brain damage either at birth or during development? Could these wild temper tantrums be temporal lobe epilepsy? An encephalogram, comprehensive IQ testing in the older child, and thorough examination of the nervous system may give some clues.

Then look at Johnny's environment. Is he reacting psychologically or physically to it? Vomiting cows' milk derivatives, screaming in pain? Is he living in an apartment in a large, unpleasant building with a trapped, lonely mother deserted by the father? Are both parents living in disharmony or in cold unresponsiveness? Does he react in the same fashion if someone else cares for him in another place? What is happening at school or in his group of playmates? Do those caring for him understand normal development, his particular problems either in communication or relating or understanding?

Once these questions have been answered, one can then determine fairly well whether this behavior is reactive in a normal psychological fashion or is psychotic or physical. This does need the experience of a practical general pediatrician; and even then it may not be possible to tell which is true until a child is six or seven years of age, but parents can be counseled in management of diet and behavior and if necessary given medication to stabilize the situation over the years. It may be possible to get the parents some sleep and help them learn to love their Jekyll-and-Hyde offspring, finding ways in which the child's needs can be met to ensure adjustment to the environment. This may even prevent the breakup of marriage. There is now quite a lot of useful educational material to help the hyperkinetic and the specific learning difficulty children. There are also many self-help groups where parents can share their problems. It is certainly not going to hurt any child to try out the Feingold diet. It is not an easy diet to follow and you will probably find that the whole family has to adhere to it accurately for at least a month to give it a fair trial. However, there is no doubt whatever that these children should be fully assessed by an experienced pediatrician. These children will then be almost certainly referred for special testing such as hearing, sight, electroencephalogram and general psychological examination. It cannot be assumed that if a parent simply survives the day-to-day living with such a child, the child will necessarily grow out of the problem. The child is going to need help, guidance, love, and understanding all the way.

16
Preventing Illness
in Your Child

The visit to the doctor is usually for some emergency or sudden illness, yet much illness is preventable and most parents are anxious to do all they can to take active measures to keep children healthy. Health is a positive thing, very different from the mere absence of disease; to quote again the definition of the World Health Organization, "Health is complete mental, social and physical well-being." The report on divine healing and cooperation between doctors and clergy goes further. It defines health as a condition of satisfactory functioning of the whole organism. It states that health, wholeness, and holiness are closely related. In other words, we should add spiritual health to the World Health Organization definition, and, in fact, I believe this was considered and was actually included in the Rights of the Child.

Parents do not want to know all about disease; I can assure you it greatly adds to your fears and worries if you do. We want to know more about health and happiness; we want to rid ourselves of fears and anxiety, and live. We want our children to live and enjoy living, and the experts tell us that their ultimate chances of health and happiness depend on their parents and the quality of home life those parents provide. Heredity or environment, which matters most? I am not getting involved in that old argument. We know that many illnesses occur in certain families, but we know more and more about their prevention. Everyone can do something about environment, so let us avoid futile argument and take a positive attitude to our task. What really matters for most children is how their parents cope with their environment and either adapt to it or change it to suit them and their family and how they show their children how to cope and what standards they teach them to live by.

Attitudes and habits

Medical science has long been telling us how important are the first five years of life in the development of a healthy body; not only does food and hygiene and the quality of care affect its development, but future health will depend on the attitudes acquired regarding diet, sleep, exercise, and cleanliness. The habits children develop in the first years of life depend on their parents. The psychiatrists have now added their piece. They say that mental health, even more than physical health, is dependent upon the treatment the child receives in the first five years. They say that in those years we lay down all our reaction patterns. Our early experiences with mother, father, brothers, and sisters will determine our ability to adjust to society and live with ourselves. Add that oft-quoted statement of the Jesuit priest who said, "Give me a child for the first seven years and anyone may teach him later." Can anyone doubt the importance of the first five years of life?

The basic family unit

I do not know how to prevent illness in children, but a few suggestions may not go astray. Despite the thoughts of "advanced" thinkers and the experiments of scientists and social reformers, we seem constantly to come back to the family unit as the basic unit in our society. It is ideally within the framework of the normal, happy, everyday family that the child's basic needs are best supplied; the needs for love and security and male and female influence are best supplied by a mother and father who love each other and are faithful to each other. These factors can triumph over the most difficult material situations. It seems to me that if we want our children to live well-adjusted lives, then we must look to the way nature intended life to be lived. That does not mean any nonsense like running around in a nudist camp or chewing up lettuce and cabbage and nuts like a lot of rabbits, nor does it mean an unrestricted outlet for basic instincts, which some so-called psychologists call nature's way. It means looking for what our minds and bodies need for full development in the society in which we live. Any happily married couple will look pityingly at the Don Juans and Casanovas trying to reconcile their middle-aged bodies with their stunted, adolescent emotional behavior, and will say what a poor thing they have compared with the mature love that develops through the ups and downs of marriage. It is too easy to be misled by Hollywood and patent medicine advertisements into a false idea of what nature does regard as necessary for our minds and bodies.

Who can help the modern parent to rear children in modern society surrounded by such queer senses of values? In a country where governments openly state that big-scale gambling is the way to raise money for opera houses and hospitals, where churches sponsor gambling, where some newspapers show astonishing little respect for the truth, and the educational system largely prepares children to earn a living, not to live and rear a family, it is not easy to keep our wits about us and think clearly. Many mothers complain bitterly that a generation of children's specialists stopped them from nursing and rocking their babies and told them to let the baby cry. Otherwise, the child would be spoiled. Could that have happened to women whose basic aim was to provide an environment that conformed with nature's requirements?

What it means to be a parent

Our first responsibility, then, is to face up to what being a parent involves, to learn what environment is necessary, and set about providing it. Nature's first and greatest requirement is undoubtedly love that provides both mental and physical security, and the family merely provides the ideal framework in which to express love. To children, love is indeed nature's second sun; it provides the warmth in which they thrive, but they must feel it and see it and hear it. How can a child believe in love if unjustly and impatiently slapped and shouted at, if the mother goes off to work whether her offspring is sick or well, if the child comes home to an empty house after school, and if the father's main idea at the weekend seems to be to get away from the children?

Have you heard the story of the enthusiastic young dairy farmer who won all the prizes in the local shows and whose cows surpassed the yield of all other cows in the district? Then he fell in love and he stopped fondling his cows and talking to them. He cared for them just as well, but when he transferred his demonstrations of affection to his girl friend, the cows became as other cows. An elderly friend of mine who grows lovely roses insists that they do better if you talk to them; well, if roses and cows respond to affection, children thrive on it. Love is their number one requirement; it needs to be a vital living force in the home, but what is it? Read the thirteenth chapter of Paul's first epistle to the Corinthians. There is nothing sanctimonious or sentimental about this; it is deadly serious, scientific fact. Love is no sickly sweet, glamorous Hollywood emotion; it is what provides security for children, and they need it to keep them well. The World Health Organization report on mental health in childhood states that "the child who feels secure is halfway to health."

What every child needs

We know that every child is different; each has a special mental and physical makeup, and what is right for one is often wrong for another. The nervous child, the allergic child, and the physically handicapped child are all individual studies, but all need the same basic home environment that gives love, encouragement, and reasonable living conditions. Children are very like plants; they need fresh air, sunlight, and a certain amount of protection while they grow; they need room to grow mentally and physically, a well-balanced diet, a certain amount of cultivation, and a certain amount of water applied externally—neither children nor plants like too much. Fresh air, exercise, and adequate rest may seem too obvious to mention, but so many avenues of entertainment available often mean that it is very easy for any child to miss the essential needs.

Protection does not mean coddling the child and allowing all that is desired. There are mothers keen on what they call child psychology who say, "My child must not be frustrated; he must develop fully and express himself," which he proceeds to do all over the walls and furniture with complete disregard for other people's rights and property. These mothers may murmur gently, "Darling, put down Mrs. Brown's pretty vase. Mommy would not like you to break it," as it crashes to the floor. Rapid removal of the vase and substitution of something unbreakable prior to the accident would have saved the vase and given the child the valuable knowledge that there are things that must be left alone. But the mother will stand by and see that her child gets something else. If a child is continually indulged, the eventual result is a sense of supreme importance, a power and infallibility that leads to a false sense of security failing to stand up to the outside world. There is no respect for parents or authority, because by fair means or foul, the child has always been able to get whatever was desired and the parents have given in regardless of moral issues. Psychiatrists tell us that there may be a breakdown when this child suddenly comes to the realization of having no true security and no standards of conduct; however, they tell us, too, that children must have a sense of power and self-importance and that they need guidance according to their stage of development. Here is where the cultivation comes in. Some need pruning more than others.

It means establishing good routines, habit training, training in elementary hygiene, good manners, and consideration for others. The child gets a better sense of security if there is a good idea of what to expect of society and the child knows it is possible to fit in. That does not mean going to extremes. Rigid feeding schedules, rigid habit training, forcing a child into the mold you want, can all result in a nervous, browbeaten child who is not self-reliant, or in a resentful, difficult child.

Like plants, children should not be coddled. Physical coddling, overclothing, overfeeding and overprotection against germs mean a soft child with poor resistance to infections. There are women who will not put a six-month old baby on the floor on a rug and who boil the water for an eighteen-month-old child and who are in fact so germ-conscious that the child gets little chance to meet the everyday bacteria in small doses and so build up immunity. Every mother longs to protect her child, but the child has to learn to go out alone and meet the pleasant and unpleasant. Children have never been spoiled by genuine love and interest in their well-being, but they can be spoiled by lavish, illogical displays of affection, super-abundance of material possessions, and ignorance of their real needs.

Diet

The importance of a good, balanced diet has already been discussed and it needs more than mere knowledge on the mother's part; it needs common sense too. There are mothers who say, "I always buy the best fillet steak and he has an orange every day, even when they are fifteen cents each, yet he has nothing to show for it." How can a doctor teach the mother in one or two short consultations that there are excellent substitutes for oranges out of season? How can we teach a woman that cheap cuts of meat can be just as nutritious as the expensive, when she believes that a thing is good because it is expensive? Mothers force milk into a child who would cheerfully eat cheese or fish soup; they pile big helpings onto a child's plate because they have no idea how much the child should eat. A child must have protective vitamins and body-building food, but I do feel sorry for the child who is not allowed desserts because of possible problems with teeth, or shellfish because they are indigestible, or mushrooms or oysters because granny got poisoned once. This is rather a negative approach; after all, they may be acquired tastes and for special occasions only, but what a serious loss to one's enjoyment of life not to know the joys of eating lobsters and oysters. It is also very difficult to get a good, balanced diet into the older child who has been allowed to develop fads. It is not so very difficult for every mother to see that her child will eat most foods by the age of eight. The secret of doing this is really no secret at all, since it is the way to teach them cleanliness, good habits, and good manners; we have to do what we expect them to do by the most effective method of teaching anything—by example. They will unconsciously copy those they love.

Do we wash too much?

Now what about water. Lovely to play in and wonderfully messy, it is good to drink but not much fun applied externally too frequently. That may sound heretical, but too many people wash out their body fats in steaming baths, and a lot of unfortunate children are too clean. By all means see that a child learns pride in appearance and looks after good clothes, but let us be reasonable about jeans, overalls, khaki shorts, and play clothes in general. What does it really matter how dirty they get? How can a child learn to climb a tree or find out how a car works without getting dirty?

When I maintain that we must find out what nature requires for health, I do not mean that we ignore modern science; far from it. In our civilized lives we are eating foods that are pleasant and nutritious and far more pleasing to our palates than those of years ago, and if they lack some vitamins, science can show us how to replace them. Science can show us some excellent shortcuts that produce the same end result that nature did less efficiently. A good example of this is immunization against such diseases as poliomyelitis, diphtheria, and tetanus, all of which should be done, for they offer a high degree of protection.

Nature does not prepare people to live in a complicated civilization; women do not know by instinct how to run a house, cook a balanced diet, or care for a baby; nature merely provides the basic urges. It is for parents to learn and apply modern scientific knowledge to the business of bringing up a family. Preparation starts before marriage, but the really effective preparation for parenthood can be done in the period of waiting for the arrival of the first baby. A mother who prepares for a natural childbirth can more confidently expect a normal labor and a baby that is far less likely to have any birth accidents than the baby of the frightened mother who demands her anesthetic early. A factor in keeping children well is certainly the sincerity with which parents prepare themselves for the task, and research work shows that this is particularly true for the mother.

Essential needs of children

Let us then summarize something of what children need for health:

1. A happy home, interested, responsible parents, reasonable discipline, a firm moral and religious code, a moderately elastic routine that gives security but allows freedom for self-expression.

2. Sunlight, fresh air, exercise, adequate rest, a balanced diet prepared by a good cook with common sense and no cranky ideas.

3. Active measures to protect them against the greatest hazards to child life, such as accident prevention and infections.

4. A positive approach to life in general. If we go looking for trouble we usually find it, and this applies to ill health too.

17
Childhood Infections and Immunization Plan

Infections are common in the early years of life. They still cause death and serious illness, though immunization has greatly reduced these hazards. It is unwise to treat infections without consulting a doctor. Even if you feel sure you know what the fever is caused by, diagnosis should be confirmed and complications prevented.

The incubation period is the time that elapses between exposure to infection and the development of signs of illness. The infectious period is the time during which the patient can infect other people.

Infections are usually caught from someone who has the disease or is a "carrier," i.e., is carrying the germ, usually in the nose or bowel or on the skin.

There are rules about isolation, the period during which a person should be kept from contact with others, and the length of time the child should be kept from school, when in contact with, or after having, the disease.

Disinfection should be considered. Though most germs die at room temperature, some, like the streptococcal and staphylococcal infections, are more resistant and require more stringent methods of control.

TABLE OF INFECTIONS

Infection	Incubation Period (days)	Infectious Period	Symptoms	Prevention
Chicken pox	14–21	From day before rash to scabs healed.	Red spots, blisters, scabs.	None.
Diphtheria	2–10	Onset to 4 weeks.	Sore throat, difficulty swallowing, fever.	Immunization with triple antigen.
Gastroenteritis	1	While any symptoms are present.	Vomiting, offensive loose bowel movements that may contain blood, mucus.	Good hygiene
German measles	14–21	Before rash to 4–5 days after appearance.	Fine rash, swollen glands.	Serum for pregnant women only.
Viral hepatitis A	15–50	Probably up to 4 weeks.	Nausea, abdominal pain, fever and jaundice, dark urine.	Gamma globulin given within 2 weeks of contact gives 6 weeks' protection. Spread is by food and drink contaminated by infectious person. Therefore, strict isolation of patient and feeding and toilet utensils.

Infection	Incubation Period (days)	Infectious Period	Symptoms	Prevention
Hepatitis B	60–150	Spread by injection of human serum or contaminated syringe. Also by excreta and close contact.	Slower onset but more severe illness than Hepatitis A.	Gamma globulin or serum within 5 days of contact, for child under 2 years, temporary; immunization, lasting.
Measles	10–12	4 or 5 days before rash to a week after.	Discharge from eyes and nose, cough, rash, red patches behind ears and on chest first, white spots in mouth	Nil.
Mumps	14–28	4–7 days before swelling till swelling subsides.	Swelling below and in front of the ears, may involve other glands.	Immunization.
Polio	7–14	2–7 days after first symptoms.	Fever, headache, paralysis.	Isolate the patient and sick pets who may be carrying it.
Ringworm	Several	Contact spread while rash present.	Scaly reddish patches—may be circular.	Avoid contact with patient, clothing, bedding, etc
Scabies	Variable (few days)	While any rash is present.	Itch worse at night; scratch marks, burrows.	

Disease	Incubation (days)	Infectious period	Symptoms	Prevention
Scarlet fever (scarlatina)	1–7	Until throat swab negative (4 weeks).	Sore throat, fine red rash—not on face.	Preventive penicillin.
Staphylococcal infection	1–4	While symptoms present.	Boils, impetigo, carbuncles.	No immunization. Use of antiseptic lotions and soaps.
Streptococcal throats	2–5	Few days before onset to end of symptoms.	Sore throat, tonsillitis.	No immunization. Preventive penicillin.
Tetanus	1–30		Wound, "lock jaw," convulsion.	Triple antigen immunization. Booster after any injury.
Whooping cough	5–21	Onset of symptoms for 4 weeks.	Spasms of coughing until purple in face, may be followed by vomiting.	Triple antigen.
Worms		While worms are present.	Pains in abdomen, irritability, itchy tail.	Good hygiene. Hand washing after toilet and before meals.

IMMUNIZATION PLAN

Age	Disease	Agent	Visit
2–3 months	Whooping cough Diphtheria Tetanus Poliomyelitis	Triple Antigen Sabin oral vaccine	1
4–5 months	Whooping cough Diphtheria Tetanus Poliomyelitis	Triple Antigen Sabin oral vaccine	2
6–7 months	Whooping cough Diphtheria Tetanus Poliomyelitis	Triple Antigen Sabin oral vaccine	3
12–15 months	Measles	Viral vaccine	4
12–24 months	Smallpox	Calf Lymph (freeze-dried)	5
18 months	Whooping cough Diphtheria Tetanus	Triple Antigen, omitting whooping cough if there was any previous reaction.	6
4–6 years	Diphtheria Tetanus* Poliomyelitis	Combined diphtheria and tetanus toxoid Sabin oral vaccine	7
12–14 years	Rubella	German Measles vaccine for girls	8

* Tetanus vaccination should be repeated at five-year intervals, but a tetanus booster is given after any penetrating injury in that interval.

Index